2. Oatmeal with Flaxseeds and Almonds

Ingredient:

• 1 cup old•fashioned oats
• 1 1/2 cups unsweetened almond milk (or milk of your choice)
• 1 tbsp ground flaxseeds
• 2 tbsp sliced almonds
• 1 tsp honey or maple syrup (optional)
• Pinch of cinnamon

Instructions:

1. In a small saucepan, combine the oats and almond milk. Bring to a simmer over medium heat, stirring occasionally.

2. Once the oats have thickened to your desired consistency, usually 5•7 minutes, remove from heat.

3. Stir in the ground flaxseeds, sliced almonds, and a pinch of cinnamon.

4. If desired, drizzle with a small amount of honey or maple syrup for a touch of sweetness.

Why this is a good option for menopause:

• Oats are a complex carbohydrate that can help provide sustained energy and keep you feeling full, which can be helpful during menopause.

• Flaxseeds are a great source of fiber, omega•3 fatty acids, and phytoestrogens, which can help manage menopausal symptoms like hot flashes and mood changes.

• Almonds are rich in healthy fats, protein, and magnesium, all of which can support bone health and overall well•being during menopause.

• Cinnamon may have anti•inflammatory properties and can help regulate blood sugar levels, which can be beneficial for menopausal women.

This warm, comforting breakfast can be a nutritious and satisfying way to start the day during the menopausal transition.

3. Avocado Toast with a Poached Egg

Ingredient:

- 2 slices of whole•grain or sourdough bread
- 1 ripe avocado, mashed
- 2 eggs
- 1 tbsp white vinegar
- Salt and pepper to taste
- Optional toppings: sliced tomatoes, sprouts, red pepper flakes, etc.

Instructions:

1. Toast the bread slices until lightly golden.

2. In a small saucepan, bring 3•4 inches of water to a gentle simmer. Add the white vinegar.

3. Crack the eggs one at a time into the simmering water, being careful not to overcrowd the pan. Poach the eggs for 3•5 minutes, until the whites are set but the yolks are still runny.

4. Remove the poached eggs from the water using a slotted spoon. Spread the mashed avocado evenly over the toasted bread slices. Top each slice of avocado toast with a poached egg. Season with salt and pepper, and any additional desired toppings.

Why this is a good option for menopause:

- Avocado is a great source of healthy fats, fiber, and antioxidants, which can help support overall health and manage menopausal symptoms.

- Eggs are a high•quality protein source that can help maintain muscle mass and bone health during menopause.

- The combination of healthy fats, protein, and complex carbohydrates from the whole•grain bread can help provide sustained energy and keep you feeling full.

- The nutrient•dense ingredients in this dish can help support overall well•being and potentially alleviate some menopausal symptoms, such as hot flashes and mood changes.

This simple, yet satisfying meal can be a great option for a nutritious breakfast or lunch during the menopausal transition.

Welcome to **_"The New Menopause Cookbook: Soothing Foods to Ease Menopause Symptoms With 115+ Recipes."_** _This book is crafted with you in mind, offering a delicious and nourishing approach to managing the often challenging symptoms of menopause._

Menopause is a significant transition in a woman's life, bringing about a host of physical and emotional changes. From hot flashes and night sweats to mood swings and sleep disturbances, the journey through menopause can sometimes feel overwhelming. However, it's also a time of transformation and empowerment, and food can play a pivotal role in making this journey smoother and more enjoyable.

In this cookbook, you will find over 115 recipes designed to support your well-being and ease menopausal symptoms. Each dish is carefully crafted to be rich in nutrients that help balance hormones, boost energy, and enhance mood. We've included a variety of recipes—from hearty breakfasts and satisfying lunches to wholesome dinners and delectable desserts—ensuring that you have tasty options for every meal of the day.

What sets this cookbook apart is its focus on ingredients that are known to support menopausal health. You'll discover the benefits of phytoestrogen-rich foods, omega-3 fatty acids, antioxidants, and vitamins that can help alleviate symptoms and promote overall wellness. Whether you're dealing with hot flashes, weight gain, or low energy, the recipes here are designed to nourish your body and help you feel your best.

We've also included practical tips on meal planning, hydration, and lifestyle choices that complement your diet, making it easier to adopt habits that support your health during this transition. Our goal is to empower you with the knowledge and tools you need to take control of your health and embrace this new chapter with confidence and grace.

So, let's embark on this culinary journey together. Whether you're an experienced cook or a kitchen novice, you'll find joy and inspiration in these pages. Here's to delicious, wholesome meals that soothe, nourish, and uplift you through every stage of menopause.

Let's get cooking!

1. Greek Yogurt with Berries and Chia Seeds

Ingredient:

• 1 cup plain Greek yogurt
• 1/2 cup mixed berries (such as blueberries, raspberries, and/or blackberries)
• 1 tbsp chia seeds

Instructions:
1. Scoop the Greek yogurt into a bowl.

2. Top the yogurt with the mixed berries.

3. Sprinkle the chia seeds over the top.

4. Enjoy!

Why this is a good option for menopause:

• Greek yogurt is high in protein, which can help maintain muscle mass and bone health during menopause.

• Berries are rich in antioxidants and phytonutrients, which can help reduce inflammation and support overall health.

• Chia seeds are a great source of fiber, omega•3 fatty acids, and other nutrients that can help manage menopausal symptoms like hot flashes and mood changes.

This simple, nutrient•dense snack or breakfast can be a great addition to a balanced diet during the menopausal transition. The combination of protein, fiber, and healthy fats can help keep you feeling full and satisfied.

4. Smoothie with Spinach, Banana, and Almond Milk

Ingredient:

• 1 cup unsweetened almond milk
• 1 cup fresh spinach leaves
• 1 ripe banana, frozen
• 1 tbsp ground flaxseeds
• 1 tsp honey (optional)
• Ice cubes (optional)

Instructions:

1. Add the almond milk, spinach, frozen banana, and ground flaxseeds to a high•speed blender.

2. Blend on high speed until the mixture is smooth and creamy, about 1•2 minutes.

3. If desired, add a teaspoon of honey for a touch of sweetness.

4. If you prefer a thicker consistency, add a few ice cubes and blend again. Pour the smoothie into a glass and enjoy!

Why this is a good option for menopause:

• Spinach is a nutrient•dense leafy green that is rich in vitamins, minerals, and antioxidants, which can help support overall health during menopause.

• Bananas are a good source of potassium, which can help regulate blood pressure and manage menopausal symptoms like hot flashes.

• Almond milk is a dairy•free, low•calorie alternative that is high in calcium, which is important for maintaining bone health during menopause.

• Flaxseeds are a great source of fiber, omega•3 fatty acids, and phytoestrogens, which can help alleviate menopausal symptoms like hot flashes and mood changes.

• The combination of these nutrient•dense ingredients can provide a quick and easy way to get a boost of energy, fiber, and essential vitamins and minerals during the menopausal transition.

This smoothie can be a refreshing and satisfying way to start the day or enjoy as a snack during menopause.

5. Quinoa Breakfast Bowl with Berries and Nuts

Ingredient:

- 1 tbsp chia seeds
- 1 tbsp honey or maple syrup (optional)
- 1/4 cup unsweetened almond milk
- Cinnamon to taste
- 1 cup cooked quinoa, cooled
- 1/2 cup mixed berries (such as blueberries, raspberries, and/or blackberries)
- 2 tbsp chopped walnuts or almonds

Instructions:

1. In a bowl, combine the cooked quinoa, mixed berries, chopped nuts, and chia seeds.

2. If desired, drizzle the honey or maple syrup over the top.

3. Pour the almond milk over the quinoa mixture and sprinkle with a dash of cinnamon. Stir gently to combine all the ingredients.

Why this is a good option for menopause:

• Quinoa is a gluten•free, high•protein grain that can help maintain muscle mass and provide sustained energy during menopause.

• Berries are rich in antioxidants, fiber, and phytonutrients that can help reduce inflammation and support overall health.

• Nuts, such as walnuts and almonds, are a good source of healthy fats, protein, and minerals like magnesium, which can help support bone health and manage menopausal symptoms.

• Chia seeds are a great source of fiber, omega•3 fatty acids, and other nutrients that can help alleviate menopausal symptoms like hot flashes and mood changes.

• The combination of complex carbohydrates, protein, fiber, and healthy fats in this breakfast bowl can help keep you feeling full and satisfied, which can be beneficial for managing weight during the menopausal transition.

This nutrient•dense and versatile breakfast bowl can be a great way to start the day during menopause, providing a balance of essential nutrients to support overall health and well•being.

6. Whole Grain Pancakes with Fresh Fruit

Ingredient:

• 1 cup whole wheat flour
• 1 tsp baking powder
• 1/4 tsp baking soda
• 1/4 tsp salt
• 1 egg

• 1 cup unsweetened almond milk (or milk of your choice)
• 1 tbsp honey or maple syrup
• 1 tsp vanilla extract
• 1 cup mixed fresh berries (such as blueberries, raspberries, and/or sliced strawberries)

Instructions:

1. In a medium bowl, whisk together the whole wheat flour, baking powder, baking soda, and salt.

2. In a separate bowl, beat the egg. Then stir in the almond milk, honey or maple syrup, and vanilla extract.

3. Pour the wet ingredients into the dry ingredients and stir just until combined (do not overmix).

4. Heat a lightly oiled non•stick skillet or griddle over medium heat.

5. Scoop about 1/4 cup of the batter onto the hot surface and cook for 2•3 minutes, or until bubbles start to form on the surface. Flip the pancake and cook for an additional 1•2 minutes, until golden brown.

7. Repeat with the remaining batter, keeping the cooked pancakes warm in a 200°F oven. Serve the whole grain pancakes warm, topped with the fresh mixed berries.

Why this is a good option for menopause:

• Whole wheat flour is a complex carbohydrate that can provide sustained energy and help manage blood sugar levels, which can be beneficial during menopause.

• Berries are rich in antioxidants, fiber, and phytonutrients that can help reduce inflammation and support overall health.

• The combination of complex carbohydrates, fiber, and protein from the eggs can help keep you feeling full and satisfied, which can be helpful for managing weight during the menopausal transition.

• This nutrient•dense breakfast can provide a boost of essential vitamins, minerals, and phytoestrogens that may help alleviate menopausal symptoms like hot flashes and mood changes.

7. Scrambled Eggs with Spinach and Tomatoes

Ingredient:

- 4 large eggs
- 1 tbsp olive oil
- 1 cup fresh spinach leaves, chopped
- 1/2 cup cherry tomatoes, halved
- 1 tbsp grated Parmesan cheese (optional)
- Salt and pepper to taste

Instructions:

1. In a small bowl, whisk the eggs together until well combined.

2. Heat the olive oil in a non•stick skillet over medium heat.

3. Add the chopped spinach to the skillet and sauté for 1•2 minutes, until slightly wilted.

4. Pour the whisked eggs into the skillet and let them sit for 30 seconds to a minute, until the bottom starts to set.

5. Using a spatula, gently push the eggs from the edge of the pan towards the center, allowing the uncooked egg to flow to the edges. Repeat this process until the eggs are mostly cooked but still slightly moist.

6. Stir in the halved cherry tomatoes and continue cooking for another 1•2 minutes, until the eggs are fully cooked.

7. Remove the skillet from heat and sprinkle the scrambled eggs with Parmesan cheese, if desired. Season with salt and pepper to taste. Serve the scrambled eggs warm.

Why this is a good option for menopause:

• Eggs are a high•quality protein source that can help maintain muscle mass and bone health during menopause.

• Spinach is a nutrient•dense leafy green that is rich in vitamins, minerals, and antioxidants, which can support overall health and potentially alleviate menopausal symptoms.

• Tomatoes are a good source of lycopene, an antioxidant that may help reduce the risk of certain health conditions associated with menopause.

• The combination of protein, fiber, and essential nutrients in this dish can help provide sustained energy and keep you feeling full, which can be beneficial for managing weight during the menopausal transition.

8. Overnight Oats with Pumpkin Seeds

Ingredient:

• 1 cup old•fashioned rolled oats
• 1 cup unsweetened almond milk (or milk of your choice)
• 2 tbsp chia seeds
• 2 tbsp pumpkin seeds
• 1 tsp honey or maple syrup (optional)
• 1/2 tsp ground cinnamon
• Pinch of salt

Instructions:

1. In a medium•sized bowl or mason jar, combine the rolled oats, almond milk, chia seeds, pumpkin seeds, honey or maple syrup (if using), cinnamon, and a pinch of salt.

2. Stir all the ingredients together until well combined.

3. Cover the bowl or seal the mason jar and refrigerate overnight, or for at least 4 hours.

4. When ready to serve, give the overnight oats a stir and enjoy them chilled or at room temperature.

Why this is a good option for menopause:

• Oats are a complex carbohydrate that can provide sustained energy and help manage blood sugar levels, which can be beneficial during menopause.

• Chia seeds are a great source of fiber, omega•3 fatty acids, and other nutrients that can help alleviate menopausal symptoms like hot flashes and mood changes.

• Pumpkin seeds are rich in magnesium, zinc, and other minerals that can support bone health and overall well•being during the menopausal transition.

• Cinnamon may have anti•inflammatory properties and can help regulate blood sugar levels, which can be helpful for menopausal women.

• The combination of protein, fiber, and healthy fats in this dish can help keep you feeling full and satisfied, which can be beneficial for managing weight during menopause.

This easy, make•ahead breakfast can be a nutritious and convenient option to start your day during the menopausal transition.

9. Cottage Cheese with Pineapple and Walnuts

Ingredient:

• 1 cup low•fat or non•fat cottage cheese
• 1/2 cup fresh pineapple, diced
• 2 tbsp chopped walnuts
• 1 tsp honey (optional)
• Pinch of cinnamon

Instructions:
1. In a bowl, combine the cottage cheese, diced pineapple, and chopped walnuts.

2. If desired, drizzle the honey over the top and sprinkle with a pinch of cinnamon.

3. Stir gently to combine all the ingredients.

4. Enjoy the cottage cheese mixture chilled or at room temperature.

Why this is a good option for menopause:

• Cottage cheese is a great source of protein, which can help maintain muscle mass and bone health during menopause.

• Pineapple is a good source of vitamin C, which can help support the immune system and potentially alleviate menopausal symptoms like hot flashes.

• Walnuts are rich in healthy fats, protein, and magnesium, all of which can support overall health and well•being during the menopausal transition.

• The combination of protein, fiber, and healthy fats in this dish can help keep you feeling full and satisfied, which can be beneficial for managing weight during menopause.

• The natural sweetness from the pineapple and the optional honey can provide a touch of sweetness without the need for added sugars.

This simple, nutrient•dense snack or light meal can be a great option for women during menopause, providing a balance of essential nutrients to support overall health and potentially alleviate menopausal symptoms.

10. Chia Seed Pudding with Mango

Ingredient:

• 1/4 cup chia seeds
• 1 cup unsweetened almond milk (or milk of your choice)
• 1 tbsp honey or maple syrup (optional)
• 1/2 tsp vanilla extract
• 1 cup diced fresh mango

Instructions:
1. In a medium•sized bowl, whisk together the chia seeds, almond milk, honey or maple syrup (if using), and vanilla extract.

2. Cover the bowl and refrigerate for at least 4 hours, or overnight, stirring occasionally, until the mixture has thickened to a pudding•like consistency.

3. When ready to serve, stir the chia seed pudding and top with the diced mango. Enjoy the chia seed pudding chilled.

Why this is a good option for menopause:

• Chia seeds are a great source of fiber, omega•3 fatty acids, and other nutrients that can help alleviate menopausal symptoms like hot flashes and mood changes.

• Almond milk is a dairy•free, low•calorie alternative that is high in calcium, which is important for maintaining bone health during menopause.

• Mango is a nutrient•dense fruit that is rich in vitamins, minerals, and antioxidants, which can support overall health and potentially reduce inflammation during the menopausal transition.

• The combination of protein, fiber, and healthy fats in this dish can help keep you feeling full and satisfied, which can be beneficial for managing weight during menopause.

• The natural sweetness from the mango and optional honey can provide a touch of sweetness without the need for added sugars.

This easy, make•ahead breakfast or snack can be a delicious and nutritious option for women during menopause, providing a balance of essential nutrients to support overall health and well•being.

11. Smoked Salmon and Avocado on Whole Grain Bread

Ingredient:

- 2 slices of whole grain bread
- 2 oz smoked salmon
- 1/2 ripe avocado, sliced
- 1 tbsp cream cheese (optional)
- 1 tsp lemon juice
- Salt and pepper to taste

Instructions:

1. Toast the whole grain bread slices until lightly golden.

2. Spread the cream cheese (if using) evenly over the toasted bread slices.

3. Layer the smoked salmon and avocado slices on top of the bread.

4. Drizzle the lemon juice over the avocado. Season with a pinch of salt and pepper.

Why this is a good option for menopause:

- Whole grain bread is a complex carbohydrate that can provide sustained energy and help manage blood sugar levels, which can be beneficial during menopause.

- Smoked salmon is a good source of protein, omega•3 fatty acids, and other nutrients that can support overall health and potentially alleviate menopausal symptoms.

- Avocado is rich in healthy fats, fiber, and antioxidants, which can help reduce inflammation and support overall well•being during the menopausal transition.

- The combination of protein, healthy fats, and complex carbohydrates in this dish can help keep you feeling full and satisfied, which can be beneficial for managing weight during menopause.

- The lemon juice can provide a refreshing and tangy flavor, while also potentially offering some anti•inflammatory benefits.

This simple, yet nutrient•dense open•faced sandwich can be a great option for a quick and satisfying breakfast or lunch during menopause.

12. Apple Cinnamon Quinoa

Ingredient:

• 1 cup uncooked quinoa, rinsed
• 2 cups unsweetened almond milk (or milk of your choice)
• 1 medium apple, peeled, cored, and diced
• 2 tsp ground cinnamon
• 1 tbsp honey or maple syrup (optional)
• 1/4 tsp ground nutmeg
• Pinch of salt

Instructions:

1. In a medium saucepan, combine the rinsed quinoa and almond milk. Bring the mixture to a boil over medium•high heat.

2. Once boiling, reduce the heat to low, cover the saucepan, and simmer for 15•20 minutes, or until the quinoa is cooked and the liquid is absorbed.

3. Remove the saucepan from the heat and stir in the diced apple, cinnamon, honey or maple syrup (if using), nutmeg, and a pinch of salt. Serve the apple cinnamon quinoa warm, or allow it to cool and enjoy it chilled.

Why this is a good option for menopause:

• Quinoa is a gluten•free, high•protein grain that can help maintain muscle mass and provide sustained energy during menopause.

• Apples are a good source of fiber, antioxidants, and phytonutrients that can help support overall health and potentially alleviate menopausal symptoms.

• Cinnamon and nutmeg are spices that may have anti•inflammatory properties and can help regulate blood sugar levels, which can be beneficial for menopausal women.

• The combination of complex carbohydrates, protein, and fiber in this dish can help keep you feeling full and satisfied, which can be helpful for managing weight during the menopausal transition.

• The natural sweetness from the apples and optional honey or maple syrup can provide a touch of sweetness without the need for added sugars.

This warm, comforting, and nutrient•dense breakfast or snack can be a great option for women during menopause, providing a balance of essential nutrients to support overall health and well•being.

13. Buckwheat Crepes with Berries

Ingredient:

- 1 cup buckwheat flour
- 1 cup unsweetened almond milk (or milk of your choice)
- 2 eggs
- 1 tbsp honey or maple syrup (optional)
- 1/4 tsp salt
- 1 cup mixed berries (such as blueberries, raspberries, and/or blackberries)
- 2 tbsp chopped walnuts or almonds (optional)

Instructions:

1. In a medium bowl, whisk together the buckwheat flour, almond milk, eggs, honey or maple syrup (if using), and salt until the batter is smooth and free of lumps.

2. Heat a non•stick skillet or crepe pan over medium heat. Lightly grease the pan with a small amount of oil or butter.

3. Pour about 1/4 cup of the batter into the pan, tilting and swirling the pan to evenly distribute the batter and create a thin crepe.

4. Cook the crepe for 1•2 minutes, or until the edges start to lightly brown and the center is set.

5. Carefully flip the crepe and cook for an additional 30 seconds to 1 minute.

6. Remove the cooked crepe from the pan and repeat the process with the remaining batter, stacking the cooked crepes on a plate.

7. To serve, place a crepe on a plate and top with a spoonful of mixed berries and a sprinkle of chopped walnuts or almonds (if using). Fold or roll the crepe and enjoy!

Why this is a good option for menopause:

- Buckwheat is a gluten•free, nutrient•dense grain that is high in fiber, protein, and antioxidants, which can help support overall health during menopause.

- Berries are rich in antioxidants, fiber, and phytonutrients that can help reduce inflammation and potentially alleviate menopausal symptoms.

This delicious and versatile crepe dish can be a great option for a satisfying breakfast or dessert during menopause, providing a balance of essential nutrients to support overall health and well•being.

14. Veggie Omelette with Whole Grain Toast

Ingredient:

- 3 eggs
- 1 tbsp olive oil
- 1/2 cup diced bell peppers

- 1/2 cup diced onions
- 1 cup spinach leaves, chopped
- 2 tbsp crumbled feta cheese (optional)
- Salt and pepper to taste
- 2 slices of whole grain bread, toasted

Instructions:

1. In a small bowl, whisk the eggs together until well combined.

2. Heat the olive oil in a non•stick skillet over medium heat.

3. Add the diced bell peppers and onions to the skillet and sauté for 2•3 minutes, until they start to soften.

4. Pour the whisked eggs into the skillet and let them sit for 30 seconds to a minute, until the bottom starts to set.

5. Using a spatula, gently push the eggs from the edge of the pan towards the center, allowing the uncooked egg to flow to the edges. Repeat this process until the eggs are mostly cooked but still slightly moist.

6. Stir in the chopped spinach and crumbled feta cheese (if using), and continue cooking for another 1•2 minutes, until the eggs are fully cooked.

7. Season the omelette with salt and pepper to taste. Serve the veggie omelette warm, accompanied by the toasted whole grain bread.

Why this is a good option for menopause:

- Eggs are a high•quality protein source that can help maintain muscle mass and bone health during menopause.

- Vegetables like bell peppers, onions, and spinach are nutrient•dense and rich in vitamins, minerals, and antioxidants, which can support overall health and potentially alleviate menopausal symptoms.

- Feta cheese is a good source of calcium, which is important for maintaining bone health during the menopausal transition.

This simple, yet nutritious omelette and toast combination can be a great option for a satisfying breakfast or brunch during the menopausal transition.

15. Protein Smoothie with Berries and Greek Yogurt

Ingredient:

• 1 cup unsweetened almond milk (or milk of your choice)
• 1/2 cup plain Greek yogurt
• 1 cup mixed berries (such as blueberries, raspberries, and/or blackberries)
• 1 scoop vanilla or unflavored protein powder
• 1 tbsp ground flaxseeds
• 1 tsp honey (optional)

Instructions:

1. Add all the ingredients to a high•speed blender.

2. Blend on high speed until the mixture is smooth and creamy, about 1•2 minutes.

3. Pour the smoothie into a glass and enjoy immediately.

Why this is a good option for menopause:

• Greek yogurt is a great source of protein, which can help maintain muscle mass and bone health during menopause.

• Berries are rich in antioxidants, fiber, and phytonutrients that can help reduce inflammation and support overall health.

• Flaxseeds are a good source of fiber, omega•3 fatty acids, and phytoestrogens, which can help alleviate menopausal symptoms like hot flashes and mood changes.

• Protein powder can help provide an additional boost of protein, which can be beneficial for maintaining muscle mass and supporting overall well•being during the menopausal transition.

• The combination of protein, fiber, and healthy fats in this smoothie can help keep you feeling full and satisfied, which can be helpful for managing weight during menopause.

• The optional honey can provide a touch of sweetness without the need for added sugars.

This nutrient•dense smoothie can be a quick and easy way to start your day or enjoy as a snack during menopause, providing a balance of essential nutrients to support overall health and well•being.

16. Kale Salad with Quinoa and Pomegranate

Ingredient:

• 4 cups chopped kale, stems removed
• 1 cup cooked quinoa, cooled
• 1/2 cup pomegranate arils
• 2 tbsp sliced almonds

• 1 tbsp olive oil
• 1 tbsp balsamic vinegar
• 1 tsp Dijon mustard
• 1 tsp honey (optional)
• Salt and pepper to taste

Instructions:

1. In a large salad bowl, combine the chopped kale, cooked quinoa, pomegranate arils, and sliced almonds.

2. In a small bowl, whisk together the olive oil, balsamic vinegar, Dijon mustard, and honey (if using).

3. Pour the dressing over the salad and toss gently to coat the ingredients evenly. Season the salad with salt and pepper to taste. Serve the kale salad immediately or refrigerate until ready to serve.

Why this is a good option for menopause:

• Kale is a nutrient•dense leafy green that is rich in vitamins, minerals, and antioxidants, which can support overall health and potentially alleviate menopausal symptoms.

• Quinoa is a gluten•free, high•protein grain that can help maintain muscle mass and provide sustained energy during menopause.

• Pomegranate arils are a good source of antioxidants and phytonutrients that can help reduce inflammation and support overall well•being.

• Almonds are rich in healthy fats, protein, and magnesium, all of which can support bone health and manage menopausal symptoms.

• The combination of complex carbohydrates, protein, fiber, and healthy fats in this salad can help keep you feeling full and satisfied, which can be beneficial for managing weight during the menopausal transition.

This vibrant and nutrient•dense salad can be a great option for a light and satisfying meal or side dish during menopause, providing a balance of essential nutrients to support overall health and well•being.

17. Spinach Salad with Strawberries and Walnuts

Ingredient:

• 5 cups fresh spinach leaves, washed and dried
• 1 cup fresh strawberries, sliced
• 1/4 cup chopped walnuts

• 2 tbsp balsamic vinegar
• 1 tbsp olive oil
• 1 tsp Dijon mustard
• 1 tsp honey (optional)
• Salt and pepper to taste

Instructions:

1. In a large salad bowl, combine the fresh spinach leaves, sliced strawberries, and chopped walnuts.

2. In a small bowl, whisk together the balsamic vinegar, olive oil, Dijon mustard, and honey (if using).

3. Pour the dressing over the salad and toss gently to coat the ingredients evenly. Season the salad with salt and pepper to taste. Serve the spinach salad immediately.

Why this is a good option for menopause:

• Spinach is a nutrient•dense leafy green that is rich in vitamins, minerals, and antioxidants, which can support overall health and potentially alleviate menopausal symptoms.

• Strawberries are a good source of vitamin C, fiber, and antioxidants, which can help reduce inflammation and support overall well•being during the menopausal transition.

• Walnuts are a great source of healthy fats, protein, and magnesium, all of which can support bone health and manage menopausal symptoms.

• The combination of complex carbohydrates, protein, fiber, and healthy fats in this salad can help keep you feeling full and satisfied, which can be beneficial for managing weight during menopause.

• The balsamic vinegar and optional honey can provide a touch of sweetness and acidity, which can complement the other flavors in the salad.

This refreshing and nutrient•dense salad can be a great option for a light and satisfying meal or side dish during the menopausal transition, providing a balance of essential nutrients to support overall health and well•being.

18. Chickpea Salad with Cucumber and Feta

Ingredient:

- 2 tbsp olive oil
- 1 tbsp lemon juice
- 1 tsp Dijon mustard
- Salt and pepper to taste

- 1 (15 oz) can of chickpeas, drained and rinsed
- 1 cup diced cucumber
- 1/4 cup crumbled feta cheese
- 2 tbsp chopped red onion
- 2 tbsp chopped fresh parsley

Instructions:

1. In a medium bowl, combine the drained and rinsed chickpeas, diced cucumber, crumbled feta cheese, chopped red onion, and chopped parsley.

2. In a small bowl, whisk together the olive oil, lemon juice, and Dijon mustard.

3. Pour the dressing over the chickpea salad and toss gently to coat the ingredients evenly.

4. Season the salad with salt and pepper to taste. Refrigerate the chickpea salad for at least 30 minutes to allow the flavors to meld. Serve the chickpea salad chilled or at room temperature.

Why this is a good option for menopause:

• Chickpeas are a good source of plant•based protein, fiber, and complex carbohydrates, which can help maintain muscle mass and provide sustained energy during menopause.

• Cucumbers are a hydrating and nutrient•dense vegetable that is rich in vitamins, minerals, and antioxidants, which can support overall health and potentially alleviate menopausal symptoms.

• Feta cheese is a good source of calcium, which is important for maintaining bone health during the menopausal transition.

• Red onion and parsley are both rich in vitamins, minerals, and antioxidants, which can help reduce inflammation and support overall well•being.

• The combination of protein, fiber, and healthy fats in this salad can help keep you feeling full and satisfied, which can be beneficial for managing weight during menopause.

This simple, yet flavorful chickpea salad can be a great option for a light and satisfying meal or snack during the menopausal transition, providing a balance of essential nutrients to support overall health and well•being.

19. Mixed Greens with Avocado and Pumpkin Seeds

Ingredient:

- 5 cups mixed greens (such as spinach, arugula, and kale)
- 1 avocado, diced
- 1/4 cup roasted pumpkin seeds
- 2 tbsp olive oil
- 1 tbsp balsamic vinegar
- 1 tsp Dijon mustard
- 1 tsp honey (optional)
- Salt and pepper to taste

Instructions:

1. In a large salad bowl, combine the mixed greens, diced avocado, and roasted pumpkin seeds.

2. In a small bowl, whisk together the olive oil, balsamic vinegar, Dijon mustard, and honey (if using).

3. Pour the dressing over the salad and toss gently to coat the ingredients evenly. Season the salad with salt and pepper to taste. Serve the mixed greens salad immediately.

Why this is a good option for menopause:

- Mixed greens, such as spinach, arugula, and kale, are nutrient·dense and rich in vitamins, minerals, and antioxidants, which can support overall health and potentially alleviate menopausal symptoms.

- Avocado is a good source of healthy fats, fiber, and antioxidants, which can help reduce inflammation and support overall well·being during the menopausal transition.

- Pumpkin seeds are a great source of zinc, magnesium, and other minerals that can support bone health and manage menopausal symptoms.

- The combination of healthy fats, fiber, and essential nutrients in this salad can help keep you feeling full and satisfied, which can be beneficial for managing weight during menopause.

This simple, yet nutrient·dense salad can be a great option for a light and satisfying meal or side dish during the menopausal transition, providing a balance of essential nutrients to support overall health and well·being.

20. Lentil Salad with Tomatoes and Basil

Ingredient:

• 1 cup cooked lentils, cooled
• 1 cup cherry tomatoes, halved
• 1/4 cup chopped fresh basil

• 2 tbsp olive oil
• 1 tbsp balsamic vinegar
• 1 tsp Dijon mustard
• 1 garlic clove, minced
• Salt and pepper to taste

Instructions:

1. In a large bowl, combine the cooked and cooled lentils, halved cherry tomatoes, and chopped fresh basil.

2. In a small bowl, whisk together the olive oil, balsamic vinegar, Dijon mustard, and minced garlic.

3. Pour the dressing over the lentil salad and toss gently to coat the ingredients evenly. Season the salad with salt and pepper to taste.

4. Refrigerate the lentil salad for at least 30 minutes to allow the flavors to meld. Serve the lentil salad chilled or at room temperature.

Why this is a good option for menopause:

• Lentils are a good source of plant•based protein, fiber, and complex carbohydrates, which can help maintain muscle mass and provide sustained energy during menopause.

• Tomatoes are a good source of lycopene, an antioxidant that may help reduce the risk of certain health conditions associated with menopause.

• Basil is a herb that is rich in vitamins, minerals, and antioxidants, which can support overall health and potentially alleviate menopausal symptoms.

• Olive oil is a healthy fat that can help reduce inflammation and support overall well•being during the menopausal transition.

• The combination of protein, fiber, and healthy fats in this salad can help keep you feeling full and satisfied, which can be beneficial for managing weight during menopause.

• The balsamic vinegar and Dijon mustard in the dressing can provide a refreshing and tangy flavor, which can complement the other ingredients in the salad.

This vibrant and nutrient•dense lentil salad can be a great option for a light and satisfying meal or side dish during the menopausal transition, providing a balance of essential nutrients to support overall health and well•being.

21. Beetroot Salad with Goat Cheese and Arugula

Ingredient:

• 1 tsp Dijon mustard
• 1 tsp honey (optional)
• Salt and pepper to taste

• 3 medium beets, roasted, peeled, and diced
• 4 cups arugula
• 1/4 cup crumbled goat cheese
• 2 tbsp olive oil
• 1 tbsp balsamic vinegar

Instructions:

1. Preheat your oven to 400°F (200°C). Wrap the beets in foil and roast for 45•60 minutes, or until tender when pierced with a fork. Allow the beets to cool, then peel and dice them.

2. In a large salad bowl, combine the diced roasted beets, arugula, and crumbled goat cheese.

3. In a small bowl, whisk together the olive oil, balsamic vinegar, Dijon mustard, and honey (if using).

4. Pour the dressing over the salad and toss gently to coat the ingredients evenly.. Season the salad with salt and pepper to taste. Serve the beetroot salad immediately.

Why this is a good option for menopause:

• Beets are a nutrient•dense root vegetable that are rich in vitamins, minerals, and antioxidants, which can support overall health and potentially alleviate menopausal symptoms.

• Arugula is a leafy green that is high in vitamins, minerals, and phytonutrients, which can also support overall well•being during the menopausal transition.

• Goat cheese is a good source of calcium, which is important for maintaining bone health during menopause.

• Olive oil is a healthy fat that can help reduce inflammation and support overall well•being.

• The combination of complex carbohydrates, protein, fiber, and healthy fats in this salad can help keep you feeling full and satisfied, which can be beneficial for managing weight during menopause.

This vibrant and nutrient•dense beetroot salad can be a great option for a light and satisfying meal or side dish during the menopausal transition, providing a balance of essential nutrients to support overall health and well•being.

22. Greek Salad with Olive Oil Dressing

Ingredient:

• 1 head romaine lettuce, chopped
• 1 cucumber, diced
• 1 pint cherry tomatoes, halved
• 1 red onion, thinly sliced
• 1 cup kalamata olives, pitted and halved
• 1 cup crumbled feta cheese
• 1/4 cup olive oil
• 2 tablespoons red wine vinegar
• 1 tablespoon lemon juice
• 1 teaspoon dried oregano
• Salt and pepper to taste

Instructions:

1. In a large salad bowl, combine the chopped romaine, diced cucumber, halved cherry tomatoes, sliced red onion, and halved kalamata olives.

2. In a small bowl, whisk together the olive oil, red wine vinegar, lemon juice, and dried oregano. Season with salt and pepper to taste.

3. Drizzle the olive oil dressing over the salad and toss gently to coat.

4. Sprinkle the crumbled feta cheese over the top of the salad.

5. Serve immediately and enjoy!

The key to this Greek salad is using high•quality, fresh ingredients and letting the simple olive oil and vinegar dressing complement the flavors. It's a light, healthy, and delicious salad perfect for any occasion.

23. Broccoli and Cranberry Salad

Ingredient:

- 4 cups broccoli florets, chopped
- 1/2 cup dried cranberries
- 1/4 cup chopped walnuts

- 2 tbsp red onion, finely chopped
- 2 tbsp plain Greek yogurt
- 1 tbsp apple cider vinegar
- 1 tsp honey (optional)
- Salt and pepper to taste

Instructions:

1. In a large bowl, combine the chopped broccoli florets, dried cranberries, chopped walnuts, and finely chopped red onion.

2. In a small bowl, whisk together the Greek yogurt, apple cider vinegar, and honey (if using).

3. Pour the dressing over the broccoli mixture and toss gently to coat the ingredients evenly. Season the salad with salt and pepper to taste.

4. Refrigerate the broccoli and cranberry salad for at least 30 minutes to allow the flavors to meld. Serve the salad chilled or at room temperature.

Why this is a good option for menopause:

• Broccoli is a nutrient•dense vegetable that is rich in vitamins, minerals, and antioxidants, which can support overall health and potentially alleviate menopausal symptoms.

• Dried cranberries are a good source of fiber, vitamin C, and antioxidants, which can help reduce inflammation and support overall well•being during the menopausal transition.

• Walnuts are a great source of healthy fats, protein, and magnesium, all of which can support bone health and manage menopausal symptoms.

• Greek yogurt is a high•protein dairy product that can help maintain muscle mass and bone health during menopause.

• The combination of fiber, protein, and healthy fats in this salad can help keep you feeling full and satisfied, which can be beneficial for managing weight during the menopausal transition.

This refreshing and nutrient•dense salad can be a great option for a light and satisfying meal or side dish during menopause, providing a balance of essential nutrients to support overall health and well•being.

24. Sweet Potato and Black Bean Salad

Ingredient:

• 2 medium sweet potatoes, peeled and diced
• 1 (15 oz) can black beans, drained and rinsed
• 1 red bell pepper, diced
• 1 cup corn kernels (fresh or frozen)
• 1/2 red onion, diced
• 2 tablespoons olive oil
• 2 tablespoons lime juice
• 1 teaspoon ground cumin
• 1/2 teaspoon chili powder
• Salt and pepper to taste
• 2 tablespoons chopped cilantro (optional)

Instructions:

1. Preheat oven to 400°F. Toss the diced sweet potatoes with 1 tablespoon of olive oil and season with salt and pepper. Spread in a single layer on a baking sheet.

2. Roast the sweet potatoes for 20•25 minutes, stirring halfway, until tender and lightly browned. Allow to cool slightly.

3. In a large bowl, combine the roasted sweet potatoes, black beans, diced bell pepper, corn, and red onion.

4. In a small bowl, whisk together the remaining 1 tablespoon olive oil, lime juice, cumin, and chili powder. Season with salt and pepper.

5. Pour the dressing over the salad and toss gently to coat.

6. Garnish with chopped cilantro, if desired.

7. Serve the sweet potato and black bean salad chilled or at room temperature. Enjoy!

This salad is packed with flavor from the roasted sweet potatoes, black beans, and zesty lime dressing. It makes a great side dish or light main course.

25. Edamame and Red Cabbage Slaw

Ingredient:

- 1 tbsp sesame oil
- 1 tsp honey (optional)
- 1 tsp Dijon mustard
- Salt and pepper to taste

- 2 cups shredded red cabbage
- 1 cup shelled edamame, cooked according to package instructions
- 1/4 cup sliced almonds
- 2 tbsp rice vinegar

Instructions:

1. In a large bowl, combine the shredded red cabbage, cooked edamame, and sliced almonds.

2. In a small bowl, whisk together the rice vinegar, sesame oil, honey (if using), and Dijon mustard.

3. Pour the dressing over the cabbage, edamame, and almond mixture, and toss gently to coat the ingredients evenly.

4. Season the slaw with salt and pepper to taste. Refrigerate the slaw for at least 30 minutes to allow the flavors to meld. Serve the edamame and red cabbage slaw chilled or at room temperature.

Why this is a good option for menopause:

- Edamame is a good source of plant•based protein, fiber, and isoflavones, which can help alleviate menopausal symptoms like hot flashes and mood changes.

- Red cabbage is a nutrient•dense vegetable that is rich in vitamins, minerals, and antioxidants, which can support overall health and potentially reduce inflammation during the menopausal transition.

- Almonds are a good source of healthy fats, protein, and magnesium, all of which can support bone health and manage menopausal symptoms.

- The combination of protein, fiber, and healthy fats in this slaw can help keep you feeling full and satisfied, which can be beneficial for managing weight during menopause.

- The rice vinegar and optional honey can provide a touch of sweetness and acidity, which can complement the other flavors in the slaw.

This refreshing and nutrient•dense slaw can be a great option for a light and satisfying side dish or a topping for grilled proteins during the menopausal transition, providing a balance of essential nutrients to support overall health and well•being.

26. Tuna Salad with Lemon and Olive Oil

Ingredient:

• 2 (5 oz) cans of tuna, drained and flaked
• 2 tbsp olive oil
• 1 tbsp lemon juice
• 1 tbsp finely chopped red onion
• 2 tbsp chopped celery
• 2 tbsp chopped parsley
• Salt and pepper to taste

Instructions:

1. In a medium bowl, combine the flaked tuna, olive oil, lemon juice, chopped red onion, chopped celery, and chopped parsley.

2. Stir the ingredients together until well mixed.

3. Season the tuna salad with salt and pepper to taste.

4. Serve the tuna salad on a bed of greens, on whole grain bread or crackers, or as a stuffing for tomatoes or avocado halves.

Why this is a good option for menopause:

• Tuna is a good source of high•quality protein, which can help maintain muscle mass and bone health during menopause.

• Olive oil is a healthy fat that can help reduce inflammation and support overall well•being during the menopausal transition.

• Lemon juice can provide a refreshing and tangy flavor, while also potentially offering some anti•inflammatory benefits.

• Onions and celery are vegetables that are rich in vitamins, minerals, and antioxidants, which can support overall health and potentially alleviate menopausal symptoms.

• Parsley is a herb that is a good source of vitamins and minerals, including vitamin K, which is important for bone health.

• The combination of protein, healthy fats, and vegetables in this tuna salad can help keep you feeling full and satisfied, which can be beneficial for managing weight during menopause.

This simple, yet flavorful tuna salad can be a great option for a quick and nutritious lunch or snack during the menopausal transition, providing a balance of essential nutrients to support overall health and well•being.

27. Roasted Veggie Salad with Tahini Dressing

Ingredient:

- 1 medium eggplant, cubed
- 1 red bell pepper, sliced
- 1 zucchini, sliced
- 1 red onion, sliced
- 2 tablespoons olive oil
- Salt and pepper to taste
- 5 oz mixed greens
- 1/4 cup crumbled feta cheese

Tahini Dressing:
- 1/4 cup tahini
- 2 tablespoons lemon juice
- 1 garlic clove, minced
- 2 tablespoons water
- 1 teaspoon honey
- Salt and pepper to taste

Instructions:

1. Preheat oven to 400°F. Toss the cubed eggplant, sliced bell pepper, zucchini, and red onion with the olive oil. Season with salt and pepper.

2. Spread the vegetables in a single layer on a baking sheet. Roast for 20•25 minutes, stirring halfway, until tender and lightly browned. Allow to cool slightly.

3. In a small bowl, whisk together all the ingredients for the tahini dressing. Add water as needed to reach a pourable consistency.

4. In a large salad bowl, combine the roasted vegetables and mixed greens. Drizzle the tahini dressing over the top and toss gently to coat.

5. Sprinkle the crumbled feta cheese over the salad. Serve the roasted veggie salad immediately.

This salad is a great option for women going through menopause for a few reasons:

- The roasted vegetables provide fiber, vitamins, and minerals that can help support overall health during menopause.

- The tahini dressing contains healthy fats and protein from the tahini, which can help balance hormones.

- The feta cheese provides calcium, which is important for bone health during menopause.

28. Farro Salad with Butternut Squash and Pecans

Ingredient:

2 tbsp balsamic vinegar
• 1 tbsp honey (optional)
• 1 tsp Dijon mustard
• Salt and pepper to taste

• 1 cup uncooked farro, cooked according to package instructions
• 2 cups diced butternut squash
• 1 tbsp olive oil
• 2 cups baby spinach or arugula
• 1/4 cup chopped pecans
• 1/4 cup dried cranberries

Instructions:

1. Preheat your oven to 400°F (200°C).

2. Toss the diced butternut squash with the olive oil and spread it out on a baking sheet. Roast for 20•25 minutes, or until the squash is tender and lightly caramelized.

3. In a large bowl, combine the cooked farro, roasted butternut squash, chopped pecans, and dried cranberries.

4. In a small bowl, whisk together the balsamic vinegar, honey (if using), and Dijon mustard.

5. Pour the dressing over the farro salad and toss gently to coat the ingredients evenly. Season the salad with salt and pepper to taste.

7. Just before serving, add the baby spinach or arugula and toss again to incorporate. Serve the farro salad warm or at room temperature.

Why this is a good option for menopause:

• Farro is a whole grain that is high in fiber, protein, and complex carbohydrates, which can provide sustained energy and help manage blood sugar levels during menopause.

• Butternut squash is a nutrient•dense vegetable that is rich in vitamins, minerals, and antioxidants, which can support overall health and potentially alleviate menopausal symptoms.

• Pecans are a good source of healthy fats, protein, and magnesium, all of which can support bone health and manage menopausal symptoms.

• Dried cranberries are a source of fiber, vitamin C, and antioxidants, which can help reduce inflammation and support overall well•being during the menopausal transition.

• The combination of complex carbohydrates, protein, fiber, and healthy fats in this salad can help keep you feeling full and satisfied, which can be beneficial for managing weight during menopause.

29. Asian Chicken Salad with Sesame Dressing

Ingredient:

• 2 boneless, skinless chicken breasts, grilled and shredded
• 4 cups mixed greens
• 1 cup shredded red cabbage
• 1 cup shredded carrots
• 1/2 cup sliced cucumber
• 1/4 cup sliced green onions
• 2 tablespoons toasted sesame seeds

Sesame Dressing:
• 2 tablespoons sesame oil
• 2 tablespoons rice vinegar
• 1 tablespoon soy sauce
• 1 tablespoon honey
• 1 teaspoon grated ginger
• 1 garlic clove, minced
• Salt and pepper to taste

Instructions:

1. In a large salad bowl, combine the shredded chicken, mixed greens, red cabbage, carrots, cucumber, and green onions.

2. In a small bowl, whisk together all the ingredients for the sesame dressing.

3. Drizzle the sesame dressing over the salad and toss gently to coat.

4. Sprinkle the toasted sesame seeds over the top of the salad.

5. Serve the Asian Chicken Salad immediately.

This salad is a great option for women going through menopause for a few reasons:

• The lean protein from the grilled chicken can help maintain muscle mass and support overall health.

• The vegetables provide fiber, vitamins, and minerals that can help alleviate some menopausal symptoms.

• The sesame dressing contains healthy fats from the sesame oil, which can help balance hormones.

• The ginger in the dressing has anti•inflammatory properties that may help reduce menopausal discomfort.

Enjoy this flavorful and nutritious salad!

30. Quinoa and Black Bean Salad with Cilantro Lime Dressing

Ingredient:

• 2 tablespoons olive oil
• 2 tablespoons lime juice
• 1 garlic clove, minced
• 1 teaspoon honey
• Salt and pepper to taste

• 1 cup uncooked quinoa, rinsed
• 1 (15 oz) can black beans, drained and rinsed
• 1 cup diced cucumber
• 1 cup diced tomatoes
• 1/2 cup diced red onion
• 1/4 cup chopped fresh cilantro

Instructions:

1. Cook the quinoa according to package instructions. Allow to cool slightly.

2. In a large bowl, combine the cooked quinoa, black beans, diced cucumber, tomatoes, red onion, and chopped cilantro.

3. In a small bowl, whisk together the olive oil, lime juice, minced garlic, and honey. Season with salt and pepper.

4. Pour the cilantro lime dressing over the quinoa and black bean salad. Toss gently to coat. Refrigerate the salad for at least 30 minutes to allow the flavors to meld. Serve chilled or at room temperature.

This quinoa and black bean salad is a great option for women going through menopause for a few reasons:

• Quinoa is a complete protein that can help maintain muscle mass and support overall health during menopause. Black beans are a good source of fiber, which can help with digestive health.

• The vegetables provide a variety of vitamins, minerals, and antioxidants that can help alleviate menopausal symptoms.

• The cilantro lime dressing contains healthy fats from the olive oil, which can help balance hormones.

• The overall nutrient•dense composition of the salad can help support overall health and well•being during this transition.

Enjoy this refreshing and nourishing quinoa and black bean salad!

31. Lentil and Vegetable Soup

Ingredient:

- 1 tablespoon olive oil
- 1 onion, diced
- 3 carrots, peeled and diced
- 3 celery stalks, diced
- Salt and pepper to taste
- 1 bay leaf
- Chopped parsley for garnish (optional)
- 3 cloves garlic, minced
- 1 cup dried brown or green lentils, rinsed
- 6 cups low•sodium vegetable or chicken broth
- 1 (14.5 oz) can diced tomatoes
- 2 cups chopped kale or spinach
- 1 teaspoon dried thyme

Instructions:

1. In a large pot or Dutch oven, heat the olive oil over medium heat. Add the diced onion, carrots, and celery. Sauté for 5•7 minutes until the vegetables are softened.

2. Add the minced garlic and sauté for an additional minute.

3. Stir in the rinsed lentils, vegetable or chicken broth, diced tomatoes, chopped kale or spinach, dried thyme, and bay leaf. Season with salt and pepper.

4. Bring the soup to a boil, then reduce the heat to low. Simmer for 30•40 minutes, or until the lentils are tender.

5. Remove the bay leaf. Taste and adjust seasoning as needed.

6. Serve the lentil and vegetable soup hot, garnished with chopped parsley if desired.

This soup is a great option for women going through menopause for a few reasons:

- The lentils are a great source of plant•based protein, fiber, and complex carbohydrates, which can help support overall health during menopause.

- The vegetables provide a variety of vitamins, minerals, and antioxidants that can help alleviate menopausal symptoms.

- The kale or spinach is rich in calcium, which is important for bone health during menopause.

- The overall nutrient•dense composition of the soup can help support overall health and well•being during this transition.

32. Chicken and Wild Rice Soup

Ingredient:

- 1 tablespoon olive oil
- 1 onion, diced
- 1 teaspoon dried thyme
- Salt and pepper to taste
- Chopped parsley for garnish (optional)

- 3 carrots, peeled and sliced
- 3 celery stalks, sliced
- 3 cloves garlic, minced
- 1 lb boneless, skinless chicken breasts, cubed
- 6 cups low•sodium chicken broth
- 1 cup wild rice, rinsed
- 1 bay leaf

Instructions:

1. In a large pot or Dutch oven, heat the olive oil over medium heat. Add the diced onion, sliced carrots, and sliced celery. Sauté for 5•7 minutes until the vegetables are softened.

2. Add the minced garlic and cubed chicken. Cook for 2•3 minutes, stirring frequently, until the chicken is lightly browned.

3. Pour in the chicken broth and add the rinsed wild rice, bay leaf, and dried thyme. Season with salt and pepper.

4. Bring the soup to a boil, then reduce the heat to low. Simmer for 45•50 minutes, or until the wild rice is tender.

5. Remove the bay leaf. Taste and adjust seasoning as needed.

6. Serve the chicken and wild rice soup hot, garnished with chopped parsley if desired.

This soup is a great option for women going through menopause for a few reasons:

- The wild rice is a whole grain that provides fiber, which can help with digestive health during menopause.

- The chicken is a lean protein that can help maintain muscle mass and support overall health.

- The vegetables provide a variety of vitamins, minerals, and antioxidants that can help alleviate menopausal symptoms.

- The overall nutrient•dense composition of the soup can help support overall health and well•being during this transition.

Enjoy this comforting and nourishing chicken and wild rice soup!

33. Tomato Basil Soup

Ingredient:

- 2 tablespoons olive oil
- 1 onion, diced
- 3 cloves garlic, minced
- 2 (28 oz) cans diced tomatoes
- 2 cups vegetable or chicken broth
- 1/4 cup fresh basil leaves, chopped
- 1 teaspoon dried oregano
- 1 bay leaf
- Salt and pepper to taste
- Heavy cream or half·and·half (optional)
- Grated Parmesan cheese for serving (optional)

Instructions:

1. In a large pot or Dutch oven, heat the olive oil over medium heat. Add the diced onion and sauté for 5·7 minutes until translucent.

2. Add the minced garlic and cook for an additional minute, stirring constantly.

3. Pour in the canned diced tomatoes and their juices, along with the vegetable or chicken broth. Stir in the chopped fresh basil, dried oregano, and bay leaf. Season with salt and pepper.

4. Bring the soup to a simmer and let it cook for 20·25 minutes, allowing the flavors to meld.

5. Remove the bay leaf. Using an immersion blender or regular blender, puree the soup until smooth.

6. If desired, stir in a splash of heavy cream or half·and·half to add a creamy texture.

7. Serve the tomato basil soup hot, garnished with grated Parmesan cheese if desired.

This classic tomato basil soup is a comforting and flavorful dish that can be enjoyed year·round. The key ingredients provide the following benefits:

- Tomatoes: Rich in lycopene, an antioxidant that may help reduce the risk of certain cancers.

- Basil: Contains anti·inflammatory properties and can help support overall health.

- Olive oil: Provides healthy monounsaturated fats that can help balance hormones.

This soup can be a great option for women going through menopause, as it is nutrient·dense and can be easily customized to individual dietary needs and preferences.

34. Butternut Squash Soup

Ingredient:

• 1 teaspoon ground cumin
• 1/2 teaspoon ground cinnamon
• 1/4 teaspoon ground nutmeg
• Salt and pepper to taste
• Chopped parsley or pepitas for garnish

• 1 medium butternut squash, peeled, seeded, and cubed (about 4 cups)
• 1 onion, diced
• 2 cloves garlic, minced
• 2 tablespoons olive oil
• 4 cups low•sodium vegetable or chicken broth

Instructions:

1. In a large pot or Dutch oven, heat the olive oil over medium heat. Add the diced onion and sauté for 5•7 minutes until translucent.

2. Add the minced garlic and cubed butternut squash. Cook for an additional 2•3 minutes, stirring frequently.

3. Pour in the vegetable or chicken broth and stir in the ground cumin, cinnamon, and nutmeg. Season with salt and pepper.

4. Bring the soup to a boil, then reduce the heat to low. Simmer for 25•30 minutes, or until the butternut squash is very soft.

5. Using an immersion blender or regular blender, puree the soup until smooth and creamy.

6. Taste and adjust seasoning as needed. Serve the butternut squash soup hot, garnished with chopped parsley or pepitas if desired.

This butternut squash soup is a nourishing and comforting dish that can be a great option for women going through menopause for a few reasons:

• Butternut squash is rich in beta•carotene, which can help support skin and eye health during menopause.

• The soup is low in calories but high in fiber, which can help with digestive health.

• The warming spices, like cinnamon and nutmeg, may help alleviate some menopausal symptoms.

• The overall nutrient•dense composition of the soup can help support overall health and well•being during this transition.

35. Miso Soup with Tofu and Seaweed

Ingredient:

• 4 cups low•sodium vegetable or chicken broth
• 2 tablespoons white or yellow miso paste
• 1 block (14 oz) firm or extra•firm tofu, cubed
• 1 cup thinly sliced shiitake mushrooms
• 1/2 cup thinly sliced green onions
• 2 tablespoons dried wakame seaweed (or other seaweed)
• 1 teaspoon grated ginger
• 1 teaspoon soy sauce (optional)
• Salt and pepper to taste

Instructions:

1. In a medium saucepan, bring the vegetable or chicken broth to a gentle simmer over medium heat.

2. In a small bowl, whisk together the miso paste with a few tablespoons of the hot broth until smooth. Pour the miso mixture back into the saucepan, stirring to combine.

3. Add the cubed tofu, sliced shiitake mushrooms, green onions, and dried wakame seaweed to the broth. Stir in the grated ginger and soy sauce (if using).

4. Simmer the soup for 5•7 minutes, allowing the flavors to meld.

5. Taste and adjust seasoning with salt and pepper as needed.

6. Serve the miso soup hot, garnished with additional green onions if desired.

This miso soup is a nourishing and comforting dish that can be a great option for those looking for a healthy meal. The key ingredients provide the following benefits:

• Miso paste: Contains probiotics that can support gut health.

• Tofu: Provides plant•based protein and is a good source of calcium.

• Shiitake mushrooms: Rich in antioxidants and immune•boosting properties.

• Wakame seaweed: High in iodine, which is important for thyroid function.

This soup is easy to make and can be a satisfying and nutritious addition to your meal rotation.

36. Minestrone Soup with Beans and Veggies

Ingredient:

• 2 tablespoons olive oil
• 1 onion, diced
• 3 carrots, peeled and diced
• 3 celery stalks, diced
• 3 cloves garlic, minced
• Salt and pepper to taste
• Grated Parmesan cheese
for serving (optional)

• 1 (15 oz) can diced tomatoes
• 4 cups low•sodium vegetable or chicken broth
• 1 (15 oz) can kidney beans, drained and rinsed
• 1 (15 oz) can cannellini beans, drained and rinsed
• 1 cup small pasta (such as ditalini or elbow macaroni)
• 2 cups chopped kale or spinach
• 1 teaspoon dried oregano
• 1 bay leaf

Instructions:

1. In a large pot or Dutch oven, heat the olive oil over medium heat. Add the diced onion, carrots, and celery. Sauté for 5•7 minutes until the vegetables are softened.

2. Add the minced garlic and sauté for an additional minute.

3. Pour in the canned diced tomatoes, vegetable or chicken broth, drained and rinsed kidney and cannellini beans, and the small pasta. Stir in the chopped kale or spinach, dried oregano, and bay leaf. Season with salt and pepper.

4. Bring the soup to a boil, then reduce the heat to low. Simmer for 20•25 minutes, or until the pasta is tender.

5. Remove the bay leaf. Taste and adjust seasoning as needed. Serve the minestrone soup hot, garnished with grated Parmesan cheese if desired.

This minestrone soup is a great option for women going through menopause for a few reasons:

• The beans provide plant•based protein and fiber, which can help support digestive and overall health.

• The vegetables, such as kale or spinach, are rich in vitamins, minerals, and antioxidants that can help alleviate menopausal symptoms.

• The broth•based soup is hydrating and can help with any fluid retention issues during menopause.

• The overall nutrient•dense composition of the soup can help support overall health and well•being during this transition.

37. Carrot Ginger Soup

Ingredient:

- 2 tablespoons olive oil
- 1 onion, diced
- 3 cloves garlic, minced
- 1 lb carrots, peeled and sliced
- 2 teaspoons grated fresh ginger
- 4 cups low·sodium vegetable or chicken broth
- 1 cup unsweetened almond milk (or regular milk)
- 1 teaspoon ground cumin
- Salt and pepper to taste
- Chopped parsley or chives for garnish (optional)

Instructions:

1. In a large pot or Dutch oven, heat the olive oil over medium heat. Add the diced onion and sauté for 5·7 minutes until translucent.

2. Add the minced garlic and grated fresh ginger. Cook for an additional minute, stirring constantly.

3. Stir in the sliced carrots and pour in the vegetable or chicken broth. Bring the soup to a simmer.

4. Reduce the heat to low and let the soup simmer for 20·25 minutes, or until the carrots are very soft.

5. Remove the pot from the heat and use an immersion blender to puree the soup until smooth and creamy. Alternatively, you can transfer the soup to a regular blender and blend in batches.

6. Stir in the unsweetened almond milk (or regular milk) and ground cumin. Season with salt and pepper to taste. Serve the carrot ginger soup hot, garnished with chopped parsley or chives if desired.

This carrot ginger soup is a great option for women going through menopause for a few reasons:

- Carrots are rich in beta·carotene, which can help support skin and eye health during menopause.

- Ginger has anti·inflammatory properties that may help alleviate some menopausal symptoms.

- The almond milk (or regular milk) provides calcium, which is important for maintaining bone health. The overall nutrient·dense composition of the soup can help support overall health and well·being during this transition.

38. Split Pea Soup

Ingredient:

- 1 tablespoon olive oil
- 1 onion, diced
- 3 carrots, peeled and diced
- 3 celery stalks, diced
- 3 cloves garlic, minced

- 1 lb dried split peas, rinsed
- 6 cups low•sodium chicken or vegetable broth
- 1 bay leaf
- 1 teaspoon dried thyme
- Salt and pepper to taste
- Chopped parsley for garnish (optional)

Instructions:

1. In a large pot or Dutch oven, heat the olive oil over medium heat. Add the diced onion, carrots, and celery. Sauté for 5•7 minutes until the vegetables are softened.

2. Add the minced garlic and sauté for an additional minute.

3. Stir in the rinsed dried split peas, chicken or vegetable broth, bay leaf, and dried thyme. Season with salt and pepper.

4. Bring the soup to a boil, then reduce the heat to low. Simmer for 45•60 minutes, stirring occasionally, until the split peas are very soft and the soup has thickened.

5. Remove the bay leaf. Use an immersion blender or regular blender to puree the soup to your desired consistency, leaving some texture if preferred.

6. Taste and adjust seasoning as needed. Serve the split pea soup hot, garnished with chopped parsley if desired.

This split pea soup is a great option for women going through menopause for a few reasons:

• Split peas are a good source of plant•based protein, fiber, and complex carbohydrates, which can help support overall health during menopause.

• The vegetables provide a variety of vitamins, minerals, and antioxidants that can help alleviate menopausal symptoms.

• The soup is hearty and comforting, which can be soothing during this transition. The overall nutrient•dense composition of the soup can help support overall health and well•being.

Enjoy this nourishing and satisfying split pea soup!

39. Mushroom Barley Soup

Ingredient:

- 1 tablespoon olive oil
- 1 onion, diced
- 3 cloves garlic, minced
- 8 oz cremini mushrooms, sliced
- Salt and pepper to taste
- Chopped parsley for garnish (optional)
- 4 cups low·sodium vegetable or chicken broth
- 1 cup pearl barley, rinsed
- 2 carrots, peeled and diced
- 2 celery stalks, diced
- 1 bay leaf
- 1 teaspoon dried thyme

Instructions:

1. In a large pot or Dutch oven, heat the olive oil over medium heat. Add the diced onion and sauté for 3·4 minutes until translucent.

2. Add the minced garlic and sliced mushrooms. Cook for an additional 5 minutes, stirring occasionally, until the mushrooms are softened.

3. Pour in the vegetable or chicken broth and add the rinsed pearl barley, diced carrots, diced celery, bay leaf, and dried thyme. Season with salt and pepper.

4. Bring the soup to a boil, then reduce the heat to low. Simmer for 30·40 minutes, or until the barley is tender.

5. Remove the bay leaf. Taste and adjust seasoning as needed. Serve the mushroom barley soup hot, garnished with chopped parsley if desired.

This soup is a great option for women going through menopause for a few reasons:

- The barley is a whole grain that provides fiber, which can help with digestive health during menopause.

- Mushrooms are a good source of antioxidants and vitamin D, which can help support the immune system and bone health.

- The vegetables provide a variety of vitamins, minerals, and phytonutrients that can help alleviate menopausal symptoms.

- The overall nutrient·dense composition of the soup can help support overall health and well·being during this transition.

Enjoy this comforting and nourishing mushroom barley soup!

40. Sweet Potato and Red Lentil Soup

Ingredient:

- 1 tablespoon olive oil
- 1 onion, diced
- 3 cloves garlic, minced
- Salt and pepper to taste
- Chopped cilantro for garnish (optional)

- 1 lb sweet potatoes, peeled and cubed
- 1 cup red lentils, rinsed
- 4 cups low•sodium vegetable or chicken broth
- 1 teaspoon ground cumin
- 1/2 teaspoon ground coriander
- 1/4 teaspoon ground turmeric

Instructions:

1. In a large pot or Dutch oven, heat the olive oil over medium heat. Add the diced onion and sauté for 5•7 minutes until translucent.

2. Add the minced garlic and sauté for an additional minute.

3. Stir in the cubed sweet potatoes, rinsed red lentils, and vegetable or chicken broth. Season with ground cumin, coriander, turmeric, salt, and pepper.

4. Bring the soup to a boil, then reduce the heat to low. Simmer for 20•25 minutes, or until the sweet potatoes and lentils are tender.

5. Using an immersion blender or regular blender, puree the soup until smooth and creamy.

6. Taste and adjust seasoning as needed. Serve the sweet potato and red lentil soup hot, garnished with chopped cilantro if desired.

This soup is a great option for women going through menopause for a few reasons:

- Sweet potatoes are a rich source of beta•carotene, which can help support skin and eye health during menopause.

- Red lentils are a good source of plant•based protein, fiber, and complex carbohydrates, which can help support overall health.

- The warming spices, like cumin and turmeric, may help alleviate some menopausal symptoms.

- The overall nutrient•dense composition of the soup can help support overall health and well•being during this transition.

41. Chicken and Kale Soup

Ingredient:

- 1 tablespoon olive oil
- 1 onion, diced
- 3 carrots, peeled and sliced
- 3 celery stalks, sliced
- 3 cloves garlic, minced
- 1 lb boneless, skinless chicken breasts, cubed
- 6 cups low•sodium chicken broth
- 2 cups chopped kale
- 1 teaspoon dried thyme
- Salt and pepper to taste
- Chopped parsley for garnish (optional)

Instructions:

1. In a large pot or Dutch oven, heat the olive oil over medium heat. Add the diced onion, sliced carrots, and sliced celery. Sauté for 5•7 minutes until the vegetables are softened.

2. Add the minced garlic and cubed chicken. Cook for 2•3 minutes, stirring frequently, until the chicken is lightly browned.

3. Pour in the chicken broth and stir in the chopped kale and dried thyme. Season with salt and pepper.

4. Bring the soup to a simmer and let it cook for 20•25 minutes, or until the chicken is cooked through and the kale is tender.

5. Taste and adjust seasoning as needed.

6. Serve the chicken and kale soup hot, garnished with chopped parsley if desired.

This soup is a great option for women going through menopause for a few reasons:

• The chicken provides lean protein, which can help maintain muscle mass and support overall health.

• Kale is a nutrient•dense leafy green that is rich in vitamins, minerals, and antioxidants, which can help alleviate menopausal symptoms.

• The vegetables, such as carrots and celery, provide additional fiber, vitamins, and minerals that can support overall well•being.

• The overall nutrient•dense composition of the soup can help support overall health and well•being during this transition.

Enjoy this comforting and nourishing chicken and kale soup!

42. Broccoli Cheddar Soup

Ingredient:

• 2 tablespoons butter
• 1 onion, diced
• 3 cloves garlic, minced
• Salt and pepper to taste
• Chopped parsley for garnish

• 4 cups low•sodium chicken or vegetable broth
• 4 cups chopped broccoli florets
• 2 carrots, peeled and diced
• 2 tablespoons all•purpose flour
• 1 cup milk
• 2 cups shredded cheddar cheese

Instructions:

1. In a large pot or Dutch oven, melt the butter over medium heat. Add the diced onion and sauté for 5•7 minutes until translucent.

2. Add the minced garlic and cook for an additional minute, stirring constantly.

3. Pour in the chicken or vegetable broth and add the chopped broccoli florets and diced carrots. Bring the soup to a simmer.

4. Reduce the heat to low and let the soup simmer for 15•20 minutes, or until the broccoli and carrots are tender.

5. In a small bowl, whisk together the all•purpose flour and milk until smooth. Slowly pour the milk mixture into the soup, stirring constantly, to thicken the soup.

6. Reduce the heat to low and stir in the shredded cheddar cheese until melted and fully incorporated.

7. Season the soup with salt and pepper to taste. Serve the broccoli cheddar soup hot, garnished with chopped parsley if desired.

This broccoli cheddar soup can be a great option for women going through menopause for a few reasons:

• Broccoli is a nutrient•dense vegetable that is high in fiber, vitamins, and antioxidants, which can help support overall health during menopause.

• The cheddar cheese provides calcium, which is important for maintaining bone health.

• The creamy, comforting nature of the soup can be soothing and satisfying.

• The overall nutrient•dense composition of the soup can help support overall health and well•being during this transition.

43. Spicy Black Bean Soup

Ingredient:

- 2 tablespoons olive oil
- 1 onion, diced
- 3 cloves garlic, minced
- 1 bay leaf
- Salt and pepper to taste
- Chopped cilantro, sour cream, and lime wedges for serving (optional)
- 2 teaspoons ground cumin
- 1 teaspoon chili powder
- 1/4 teaspoon cayenne pepper
- 2 (15 oz) cans black beans, drained and rinsed
- 4 cups low•sodium vegetable or chicken broth
- 1 (14.5 oz) can diced tomatoes

Instructions:

1. In a large pot or Dutch oven, heat the olive oil over medium heat. Add the diced onion and sauté for 5•7 minutes until translucent.

2. Add the minced garlic, ground cumin, chili powder, and cayenne pepper. Cook for 1•2 minutes, stirring constantly, to toast the spices.

3. Stir in the drained and rinsed black beans, vegetable or chicken broth, diced tomatoes, and bay leaf. Season with salt and pepper.

4. Bring the soup to a simmer and let it cook for 20•25 minutes, allowing the flavors to meld.

5. Remove the bay leaf. Use an immersion blender or regular blender to puree about half of the soup, leaving some texture.

6. Taste and adjust seasoning as needed, adding more cayenne pepper for extra spice if desired. Serve the spicy black bean soup hot, garnished with chopped cilantro, a dollop of sour cream, and a squeeze of fresh lime juice if desired.

This spicy black bean soup can be a great option for women going through menopause for a few reasons:

• Black beans are a good source of plant•based protein, fiber, and complex carbohydrates, which can help support overall health.

• The spices, like cumin and cayenne, have anti•inflammatory properties that may help alleviate some menopausal symptoms.

• The soup is hearty and satisfying, which can be comforting during this transition. The overall nutrient•dense composition of the soup can help support overall health and well•being.

44. Zucchini and Basil Soup

Ingredient:

• 2 tablespoons olive oil
• 1 onion, diced
• 3 cloves garlic, minced
• 3 medium zucchini, diced (about 4 cups)

• 4 cups low•sodium vegetable or chicken broth
• 1/2 cup fresh basil leaves, chopped
• 1 teaspoon lemon juice
• Salt and pepper to taste
• Croutons or crushed crackers for serving (optional)

Instructions:

1. In a large pot or Dutch oven, heat the olive oil over medium heat. Add the diced onion and sauté for 5•7 minutes until translucent.

2. Add the minced garlic and sauté for an additional minute.

3. Stir in the diced zucchini and pour in the vegetable or chicken broth. Bring the soup to a simmer.

4. Reduce the heat to low and let the soup simmer for 15•20 minutes, or until the zucchini is very soft.

5. Remove the pot from the heat and use an immersion blender to puree the soup until smooth and creamy. Alternatively, you can transfer the soup to a regular blender and blend in batches.

6. Stir in the chopped fresh basil and lemon juice. Season with salt and pepper to taste.

7. Serve the zucchini and basil soup hot, garnished with croutons or crushed crackers if desired.

This zucchini and basil soup is a great option for women going through menopause for a few reasons:

• Zucchini is a low•calorie, high•fiber vegetable that can help with digestive health and weight management during menopause.

• Basil is a herb that contains anti•inflammatory properties, which may help alleviate some menopausal symptoms.

• The soup is light and easy to digest, making it a nourishing and comforting meal.The overall nutrient•dense composition of the soup can help support overall health and well•being during this transition.

45. Quinoa and Spinach Soup

Ingredient:

- 1 tablespoon olive oil
- 1 onion, diced
- 3 cloves garlic, minced
- 1 cup uncooked quinoa, rinsed
- 6 cups low•sodium vegetable or chicken broth
- 1 (15 oz) can diced tomatoes
- 2 cups fresh spinach, chopped
- 1 teaspoon dried oregano
- Salt and pepper to taste
- Grated Parmesan cheese for serving (optional)

Instructions:

1. In a large pot or Dutch oven, heat the olive oil over medium heat. Add the diced onion and sauté for 5•7 minutes until translucent.

2. Add the minced garlic and sauté for an additional minute.

3. Stir in the rinsed quinoa, vegetable or chicken broth, and diced tomatoes. Bring the soup to a boil.

4. Reduce the heat to low, cover, and simmer for 15•20 minutes, or until the quinoa is tender.

5. Stir in the chopped fresh spinach and dried oregano. Cook for an additional 2•3 minutes, or until the spinach is wilted.

6. Season the soup with salt and pepper to taste. Serve the quinoa and spinach soup hot, garnished with grated Parmesan cheese if desired.

This soup is a great option for women going through menopause for a few reasons:

- Quinoa is a complete protein that can help maintain muscle mass and support overall health during menopause.

- Spinach is a nutrient•dense leafy green that is rich in vitamins, minerals, and antioxidants, which can help alleviate menopausal symptoms.

- The overall nutrient•dense composition of the soup can help support overall health and well•being during this transition.

The combination of protein, fiber, and vitamins in this quinoa and spinach soup makes it a nourishing and comforting meal for women going through menopause. Enjoy this delicious and easy•to•prepare soup!

46. Grilled Salmon with Quinoa and Asparagus

Ingredient:

• 4 salmon fillets (about 4•6 oz each)
• 1 cup uncooked quinoa, rinsed
• 2 cups low•sodium chicken or vegetable broth

• 1 lb asparagus, trimmed
• 2 tablespoons olive oil, divided
• 1 tablespoon lemon juice
• 1 teaspoon grated lemon zest
• Salt and pepper to taste

Instructions:

1. Preheat your grill or grill pan to medium•high heat.

2. In a medium saucepan, combine the rinsed quinoa and broth. Bring to a boil, then reduce heat to low, cover, and simmer for 15•20 minutes, until the quinoa is tender and the liquid is absorbed. Fluff with a fork and set aside.

3. Toss the trimmed asparagus with 1 tablespoon of the olive oil, salt, and pepper.

4. Grill the salmon fillets for 4•6 minutes per side, or until cooked through and flaky.

5. Grill the asparagus for 3•5 minutes, turning occasionally, until tender•crisp.

6. In a small bowl, whisk together the remaining 1 tablespoon of olive oil, lemon juice, and lemon zest.

7. Serve the grilled salmon on a bed of the cooked quinoa, topped with the grilled asparagus. Drizzle the lemon•olive oil mixture over the top.

This grilled salmon dish is a great option for women going through menopause for a few reasons:

• Salmon is a rich source of omega•3 fatty acids, which can help balance hormones and support heart health.

• Quinoa is a complete protein that can help maintain muscle mass and support overall health.

• Asparagus is a nutrient•dense vegetable that provides fiber, vitamins, and minerals to support overall well•being.

• The overall nutrient•dense composition of the dish can help support overall health and well•being during this transition.

Enjoy this delicious and healthy grilled salmon, quinoa, and asparagus meal!

47. Baked Chicken Breast with Sweet Potatoes and Green Beans

Ingredient:

• 4 boneless, skinless chicken breasts
• 2 medium sweet potatoes, peeled and cubed
• 1 lb green beans, trimmed
• 2 tablespoons olive oil
• 1 teaspoon dried thyme
• 1 teaspoon paprika
• Salt and pepper to taste

Instructions:

1. Preheat your oven to 400°F. Lightly grease a large baking sheet or rimmed baking dish.

2. Place the chicken breasts, cubed sweet potatoes, and trimmed green beans on the prepared baking sheet. Drizzle with the olive oil and sprinkle with the dried thyme, paprika, salt, and pepper. Toss to coat everything evenly.

3. Bake for 25•30 minutes, or until the chicken is cooked through (internal temperature reaches 165°F) and the sweet potatoes are tender.

4. Serve the baked chicken breast with the roasted sweet potatoes and green beans.

This dish is a great option for women going through menopause for a few reasons:

• Chicken breast is a lean protein that can help maintain muscle mass and support overall health during menopause.

• Sweet potatoes are rich in beta•carotene, which can help support skin and eye health.

• Green beans are a good source of fiber, vitamins, and minerals that can help with digestive health and overall well•being.

• The overall nutrient•dense composition of the dish can help support overall health and well•being during this transition.

The combination of protein, complex carbohydrates, and fiber•rich vegetables makes this a well•balanced and nourishing meal for women going through menopause. Enjoy this delicious and easy•to•prepare baked chicken and vegetable dish!

48. Stir-Fried Tofu with Vegetables

Ingredient:

• 1 tablespoon rice vinegar
• 1 teaspoon honey
• Salt and pepper to taste
• Chopped green onions and sesame seeds for garnish (optional)

• 1 block (14 oz) extra•firm tofu, pressed and cubed
• 2 tablespoons sesame oil, divided
• 2 cups mixed vegetables (such as broccoli, bell peppers, snow peas, carrots)
• 2 cloves garlic, minced
• 1 tablespoon grated fresh ginger
• 2 tablespoons low•sodium soy sauce

Instructions:

1. In a large skillet or wok, heat 1 tablespoon of sesame oil over medium•high heat. Add the cubed tofu and stir•fry for 5•7 minutes, or until lightly browned on all sides. Transfer the tofu to a plate and set aside.

2. In the same skillet or wok, heat the remaining 1 tablespoon of sesame oil. Add the mixed vegetables and stir•fry for 3•5 minutes, or until they are crisp•tender.

3. Add the minced garlic and grated ginger to the vegetables and cook for an additional minute, stirring constantly.

4. In a small bowl, whisk together the soy sauce, rice vinegar, and honey.

5. Add the cooked tofu back to the skillet or wok, and pour the soy sauce mixture over the top. Toss everything together and cook for 2•3 minutes, or until the sauce has thickened slightly.

6. Season the stir•fried tofu and vegetables with salt and pepper to taste. Serve the stir•fry hot, garnished with chopped green onions and sesame seeds if desired. Enjoy over steamed rice or quinoa.

This stir•fried tofu dish is a great option for women going through menopause for a few reasons:

• Tofu is a plant•based protein that can help maintain muscle mass and support overall health during menopause.

• The vegetables provide a variety of vitamins, minerals, and antioxidants that can help alleviate menopausal symptoms. The ginger and soy sauce have anti•inflammatory properties that may help reduce discomfort.

• The overall nutrient•dense composition of the dish can help support overall health and well•being during this transition.

49. Quinoa Stuffed Bell Peppers

Ingredient:

- 1/4 cup chopped fresh parsley
- 2 cloves garlic, minced
- 1 teaspoon ground cumin
- Salt and pepper to taste

- 4 bell peppers (any color), halved lengthwise and seeds removed
- 1 cup cooked quinoa
- 1 (15 oz) can black beans, drained and rinsed
- 1 cup diced tomatoes
- 1/2 cup crumbled feta cheese

Instructions:

1. Preheat your oven to 375°F.

2. Arrange the bell pepper halves in a baking dish or on a rimmed baking sheet.

3. In a medium bowl, combine the cooked quinoa, black beans, diced tomatoes, feta cheese, chopped parsley, minced garlic, and ground cumin. Season with salt and pepper.

4. Spoon the quinoa mixture evenly into the bell pepper halves.

5. Cover the baking dish or sheet with foil and bake for 25•30 minutes, or until the peppers are tender.

6. Remove the foil and bake for an additional 5•10 minutes, or until the tops are lightly browned. Serve the quinoa stuffed bell peppers warm.

This dish is a great option for women going through menopause for a few reasons:

• Quinoa is a complete protein that can help maintain muscle mass and support overall health during menopause. Black beans are a good source of fiber, which can help with digestive health.

• The bell peppers provide a variety of vitamins, minerals, and antioxidants that can help alleviate menopausal symptoms. The feta cheese is a source of calcium, which is important for bone health during menopause.

• The overall nutrient•dense composition of the dish can help support overall health and well•being during this transition.

Enjoy these delicious and nourishing quinoa stuffed bell peppers!

50. Turkey and Spinach Meatballs with Marinara Sauce

Ingredient:

- 1 lb ground turkey
- 1 cup fresh spinach, finely chopped
- 1/2 cup breadcrumbs
- 1/4 cup grated Parmesan cheese
- 1 egg
- 2 cloves garlic, minced
- 1 tsp dried oregano
- 1/2 tsp salt
- 1/4 tsp black pepper

For the Marinara Sauce:
- 1 tbsp olive oil
- 1 onion, diced
- 3 cloves garlic, minced
- 1 (28 oz) can crushed tomatoes
- 1 tsp dried basil
- 1/2 tsp dried oregano
- Salt and pepper to taste

Instructions:

1. Preheat oven to 400°F. Line a baking sheet with parchment paper.

2. In a large bowl, combine the ground turkey, spinach, breadcrumbs, Parmesan, egg, garlic, oregano, salt, and pepper. Mix well until fully incorporated.

3. Roll the mixture into 1•inch meatballs and place them on the prepared baking sheet.

4. Bake for 20•25 minutes, or until the meatballs are cooked through and lightly browned.

5. While the meatballs are baking, prepare the marinara sauce. In a saucepan, heat the olive oil over medium heat. Add the onion and garlic, and sauté for 2•3 minutes until fragrant.

6. Add the crushed tomatoes, basil, oregano, and season with salt and pepper to taste. Simmer the sauce for 10•15 minutes, stirring occasionally.

7. Serve the baked meatballs with the warm marinara sauce. Enjoy!

This recipe is a good option for women going through menopause as it is high in protein from the turkey, and the spinach provides important nutrients like iron, calcium, and magnesium, which can help support bone health and overall well•being during this transition.

51. Shrimp and Broccoli Stir•Fry

Ingredient:

- 1 lb large shrimp, peeled and deveined
- 3 cups broccoli florets
- 2 tbsp olive oil
- 3 cloves garlic, minced
- 1 tbsp grated fresh ginger
- 1/4 cup low•sodium soy sauce
- 2 tbsp rice vinegar
- 1 tbsp honey
- 1 tsp sesame oil
- 1/4 tsp red pepper flakes (optional)
- Salt and pepper to taste
- Cooked brown rice, for serving

Instructions:

1. In a small bowl, whisk together the soy sauce, rice vinegar, honey, sesame oil, and red pepper flakes (if using). Set aside.

2. Heat the olive oil in a large skillet or wok over high heat. Add the garlic and ginger and cook for 30 seconds, stirring constantly, until fragrant.

3. Add the shrimp and broccoli to the skillet. Stir•fry for 3•4 minutes, or until the shrimp are partially cooked and the broccoli is crisp•tender.

4. Pour the soy sauce mixture into the skillet and bring to a simmer. Cook for 2•3 minutes, or until the shrimp are fully cooked and the sauce has thickened slightly.

5. Season with salt and pepper to taste. Serve the shrimp and broccoli stir•fry over cooked brown rice.

This dish is a great option for women during menopause for a few reasons:

1. Shrimp is a lean protein that is low in calories and high in nutrients like selenium, which can help support thyroid function.

2. Broccoli is a nutrient•dense vegetable that is high in fiber, vitamins, and minerals, including calcium, which is important for bone health during menopause.

3. The stir•fry cooking method helps to preserve the nutrients in the vegetables, and the soy sauce and ginger provide additional anti•inflammatory benefits.

52. Lentil and Veggie Shepherd's Pie

Ingredient:

For the Filling:
• 1 cup brown or green lentils, rinsed
• 3 cups vegetable broth
• 1 tbsp olive oil
• 1 onion, diced
• 3 carrots, peeled and diced
• 3 celery stalks, diced
• 3 cloves garlic, minced
• 1 tsp dried thyme
• 1 tsp dried rosemary
• 1 tsp Worcestershire sauce (use a vegetarian/vegan version if desired)
• Salt and pepper to taste

For the Topping:
• 3 medium potatoes, peeled and cubed
• 1/4 cup unsweetened almond milk (or regular milk)
• 2 tbsp butter or olive oil
• Salt and pepper to taste

Instructions:

1. Preheat your oven to 375°F (190°C).

2. In a medium saucepan, combine the lentils and vegetable broth. Bring to a boil, then reduce heat and simmer for 20•25 minutes, or until the lentils are tender. Drain any excess liquid and set aside.

3. In a large skillet, heat the olive oil over medium heat. Add the onion, carrots, and celery. Sauté for 5•7 minutes, or until the vegetables are softened.

4. Add the garlic, thyme, rosemary, Worcestershire sauce, and the cooked lentils. Season with salt and pepper to taste. Stir to combine and cook for an additional 2•3 minutes.

5. Transfer the lentil and veggie mixture to a 9•inch pie dish or baking dish.

6. In a medium saucepan, cover the cubed potatoes with water and bring to a boil. Reduce heat and simmer for 15•20 minutes, or until the potatoes are tender. Drain the potatoes and mash them with the almond milk and butter or olive oil. Season with salt and pepper. Spread the mashed potatoes evenly over the lentil and veggie mixture.

7. Bake the shepherd's pie for 25•30 minutes, or until the potatoes are lightly browned and the filling is bubbling. Let the pie cool for 5•10 minutes before serving.

This lentil and veggie shepherd's pie is a great option for women during menopause as it is high in fiber, protein, and complex carbohydrates, which can help support overall health and well•being. The vegetables and herbs also provide important nutrients and antioxidants.

53. Black Bean and Sweet Potato Enchiladas

Ingredient:

For the Filling:
• 1 medium sweet potato, peeled and diced
• 1 tbsp olive oil
• 1 onion, diced
• 3 cloves garlic, minced
• 1 (15 oz) can black beans, rinsed and drained
• 1 tsp ground cumin
• 1 tsp chili powder
• 1/2 tsp dried oregano
• Salt and pepper to taste

For the Enchilada Sauce:
• 1 (15 oz) can tomato sauce
• 1 cup low•sodium vegetable broth
• 2 tbsp chili powder
• 1 tsp ground cumin
• 1/2 tsp garlic powder
• 1/4 tsp cayenne pepper (optional)
• Salt and pepper to taste

For Assembly:
• 8•10 corn tortillas
• 1 cup shredded cheddar or
Monterey Jack cheese (optional)

Instructions:

1. Preheat your oven to 375°F (190°C).

2. In a large skillet, heat the olive oil over medium heat. Add the diced sweet potato and sauté for 5•7 minutes, or until the sweet potato is tender.

3. Add the onion and garlic to the skillet and sauté for an additional 2•3 minutes, until the onion is translucent.

4. Stir in the black beans, cumin, chili powder, and oregano. Season with salt and pepper to taste. Remove from heat and set aside.

5. In a medium saucepan, whisk together the tomato sauce, vegetable broth, chili powder, cumin, garlic powder, and cayenne pepper (if using). Bring the sauce to a simmer and cook for 5•7 minutes, stirring occasionally, until slightly thickened. Season with salt and pepper to taste.

6. Spread a thin layer of the enchilada sauce in the bottom of a 9x13 inch baking dish.

7. Warm the corn tortillas according to package instructions. Spoon a portion of the black bean and sweet potato filling onto each tortilla, then roll them up and place them seam•side down in the prepared baking dish.

8. Pour the remaining enchilada sauce over the rolled enchiladas, and sprinkle with the shredded cheese, if using.

9. Bake the enchiladas for 20•25 minutes, or until the cheese is melted and the sauce is bubbling. Serve the enchiladas warm, garnished with any desired toppings such as diced avocado, chopped cilantro, or a dollop of plain Greek yogurt

54. Baked Cod with Lemon and Dill

Ingredient:

- 1 lb cod fillets
- 2 tablespoons olive oil
- 2 tablespoons lemon juice
- 2 tablespoons chopped fresh dill
- 1 teaspoon grated lemon zest
- Salt and pepper to taste
- Lemon wedges for serving

Instructions:

1. Preheat your oven to 400°F. Lightly grease a baking dish or line it with parchment paper.

2. Place the cod fillets in the prepared baking dish.

3. In a small bowl, whisk together the olive oil, lemon juice, chopped dill, and lemon zest. Season with salt and pepper.

4. Drizzle the lemon•dill mixture over the cod fillets, making sure to evenly coat the fish.

5. Bake the cod for 15•20 minutes, or until it flakes easily with a fork and is opaque throughout.

6. Serve the baked cod immediately, garnished with lemon wedges.

This baked cod dish is a great option for women going through menopause for a few reasons:

1. Cod is a lean, high•protein fish that can help maintain muscle mass and support overall health during menopause.

2. Lemon and dill are both rich in antioxidants and have anti•inflammatory properties, which may help alleviate some menopausal symptoms.

3. The dish is low in calories and high in healthy omega•3 fatty acids, which can help balance hormones and support heart health.

4. The overall nutrient•dense composition of the dish can help support overall health and well•being during this transition.

55. Spaghetti Squash with Marinara Sauce

Ingredient:

For the Spaghetti Squash:
• 1 medium spaghetti squash,
halved lengthwise and seeds removed
• 1 tbsp olive oil
• Salt and pepper to taste

Optional Toppings:
• Grated Parmesan cheese
• Chopped fresh basil or parsley

For the Marinara Sauce:
• 1 tbsp olive oil
• 1 onion, diced
• 3 cloves garlic, minced
• 1 (28 oz) can crushed tomatoes
• 2 tbsp tomato paste
• 1 tsp dried basil
• 1 tsp dried oregano
• 1/4 tsp red pepper flakes (optional)
• Salt and pepper to taste

Instructions:

1. Preheat your oven to 400°F (200°C).

2. Place the spaghetti squash halves cut•side up on a baking sheet. Drizzle with the olive oil and season with salt and pepper.

3. Roast the spaghetti squash for 40•50 minutes, or until it's tender and easily shreds with a fork.

4. While the spaghetti squash is roasting, prepare the marinara sauce. In a medium saucepan, heat the olive oil over medium heat. Add the diced onion and sauté for 5•7 minutes, until translucent.

5. Add the minced garlic and sauté for an additional 1•2 minutes, until fragrant.

6. Stir in the crushed tomatoes, tomato paste, dried basil, dried oregano, and red pepper flakes (if using). Season with salt and pepper to taste.

7. Bring the marinara sauce to a simmer and let it cook for 10•15 minutes, stirring occasionally, to allow the flavors to meld.

8. Once the spaghetti squash is cooked, use a fork to shred the flesh into spaghetti•like strands. Serve the spaghetti squash strands topped with the warm marinara sauce. Garnish with grated Parmesan cheese and chopped fresh basil or parsley, if desired.

This spaghetti squash with marinara sauce is a great option for women during menopause as it is low in calories, high in fiber, and provides a good source of vitamins and minerals, including vitamin C, vitamin A, and potassium. The spaghetti squash also offers a lower•carb alternative to traditional pasta.

56. Grilled Portobello Mushrooms with Quinoa

Ingredient:

For the Mushrooms:
• 4 large portobello mushroom caps,
stems removed
• 2 tbsp olive oil
• 2 tbsp balsamic vinegar
• 2 cloves garlic, minced
• 1 tsp dried thyme
• Salt and pepper to taste

For the Quinoa:
• 1 cup uncooked quinoa, rinsed
• 2 cups low•sodium vegetable broth
• 1/4 cup chopped fresh parsley
• 2 tbsp lemon juice
• Salt and pepper to taste

Optional Toppings:
• Crumbled feta cheese
• Chopped fresh basil or parsley

Instructions:

1. Preheat your grill or grill pan to medium•high heat.

2. In a shallow dish, whisk together the olive oil, balsamic vinegar, garlic, and thyme. Season with salt and pepper.

3. Add the portobello mushroom caps to the dish and turn to coat them evenly in the marinade. Grill the mushrooms for 4•5 minutes per side, or until they are tender and slightly charred.

4. While the mushrooms are grilling, prepare the quinoa. In a medium saucepan, combine the rinsed quinoa and vegetable broth. Bring the mixture to a boil, then reduce the heat to low, cover, and simmer for 15•20 minutes, or until the quinoa is tender and the liquid is absorbed.

5. Fluff the cooked quinoa with a fork and stir in the chopped parsley and lemon juice. Season with salt and pepper to taste. Serve the grilled portobello mushrooms on a bed of the prepared quinoa. Top with crumbled feta cheese and chopped fresh basil or parsley, if desired.

This grilled portobello and quinoa dish is an excellent choice for women during menopause for several reasons:

• Portobello mushrooms are a good source of antioxidants, such as selenium, which can help support overall health during menopause.

• Quinoa is a nutrient•dense grain that is high in protein, fiber, and complex carbohydrates, providing sustained energy.

• The combination of the mushrooms and quinoa creates a satisfying and balanced meal that is low in calories and high in important vitamins and minerals.

57. Eggplant Parmesan (baked)

Ingredient:

• 2 medium eggplants, sliced into 1/2•inch thick rounds
• 2 eggs, beaten
• 1 cup breadcrumbs
• 1 cup grated Parmesan cheese, divided
• 2 cups marinara sauce
• 2 cups shredded mozzarella cheese
• Fresh basil leaves for garnish (optional)

Instructions:

1. Preheat your oven to 375°F. Lightly grease a 9x13 inch baking dish.

2. Dip the eggplant slices in the beaten eggs, then coat them in the breadcrumb and 1/2 cup of the Parmesan cheese mixture.

3. Arrange the breaded eggplant slices in a single layer in the prepared baking dish.

4. Bake for 20•25 minutes, flipping the slices halfway, until the eggplant is tender and the breading is golden brown.

5. Remove the baked eggplant slices from the oven and top them with the marinara sauce, mozzarella cheese, and the remaining 1/2 cup of Parmesan cheese.

6. Return the dish to the oven and bake for an additional 15•20 minutes, or until the cheese is melted and bubbly.

7. Garnish the baked eggplant Parmesan with fresh basil leaves, if desired. Serve hot and enjoy!

This baked eggplant Parmesan dish is a great option for women going through menopause for a few reasons:

• Eggplant is a low•calorie, high•fiber vegetable that can help with weight management and digestive health during menopause. The Parmesan cheese provides calcium, which is important for maintaining bone health.

• The marinara sauce is a good source of lycopene, an antioxidant that may help reduce the risk of certain cancers. The overall nutrient•dense composition of the dish can help support overall health and well•being during this transition.

58. Chickpea and Spinach Curry

Ingredient:

- 1 tbsp olive oil
- 1 onion, diced
- 3 cloves garlic, minced
- 1 tbsp grated fresh ginger
- 1 tsp ground cumin
- 1 tsp ground coriander
- 1 tsp garam masala
- 1/4 tsp cayenne pepper (optional)
- 1 (15 oz) can chickpeas, rinsed and drained
- 1 (14 oz) can diced tomatoes
- 1 cup low•sodium vegetable broth
- 1/2 tsp turmeric
- 5 oz fresh spinach, roughly chopped
- 1/4 cup full•fat coconut milk
- Salt and pepper to taste
- Chopped cilantro for garnish (optional)

Instructions:

1. In a large skillet or saucepan, heat the olive oil over medium heat. Add the diced onion and sauté for 5•7 minutes, until translucent.

2. Add the minced garlic and grated ginger to the pan and cook for 1•2 minutes, until fragrant.

3. Stir in the ground cumin, coriander, garam masala, turmeric, and cayenne pepper (if using). Cook for 1 minute, stirring constantly, to toast the spices.

4. Add the rinsed and drained chickpeas, diced tomatoes, and vegetable broth to the pan. Bring the mixture to a simmer and let it cook for 10•15 minutes, allowing the flavors to meld.

5. Stir in the chopped spinach and coconut milk. Cook for an additional 5 minutes, or until the spinach is wilted and the curry has thickened slightly.

6. Season the curry with salt and pepper to taste. Serve the chickpea and spinach curry over cooked basmati rice or with naan bread. Garnish with chopped cilantro, if desired.

This chickpea and spinach curry is an excellent choice for women during menopause for several reasons:

• Chickpeas are a great source of plant•based protein, fiber, and complex carbohydrates, which can help provide sustained energy.

• Spinach is rich in vitamins, minerals, and antioxidants, including calcium, which is important for bone health during menopause.

• The blend of warming spices, such as cumin, coriander, and turmeric, can help support overall well•being and reduce inflammation. The coconut milk adds a creamy texture and healthy fats to the dish.

59. Chicken and Veggie Skewers

Ingredient:

- 2 tbsp lemon juice
- 2 tsp dried oregano
- 1 tsp garlic powder
- 1/2 tsp salt
- 1/4 tsp black pepper

- 1 lb boneless, skinless chicken breasts, cut into 1•inch cubes
- 1 red bell pepper, cut into 1•inch pieces
- 1 yellow bell pepper, cut into 1•inch pieces
- 1 zucchini, cut into 1•inch rounds
- 1 red onion, cut into 1•inch pieces
- 2 tbsp olive oil

For Serving:
- Lemon wedges
- Chopped fresh parsley (optional)

Instructions:

1. In a large bowl, combine the cubed chicken, bell pepper pieces, zucchini rounds, and red onion pieces.

2. In a small bowl, whisk together the olive oil, lemon juice, oregano, garlic powder, salt, and black pepper.

3. Pour the marinade over the chicken and vegetables and toss to coat everything evenly. Cover the bowl and refrigerate for at least 30 minutes, or up to 4 hours.

4. Preheat your grill or grill pan to medium•high heat.

5. Thread the marinated chicken and vegetables onto skewers, alternating the ingredients.

6. Grill the skewers for 12•15 minutes, turning occasionally, until the chicken is cooked through and the vegetables are tender. Serve the chicken and veggie skewers warm, with lemon wedges and chopped fresh parsley (if using) on the side.

This dish is a great option for women during menopause for several reasons:

- Chicken is a lean protein that can help support muscle mass and overall health. The variety of vegetables, such as bell peppers, zucchini, and onions, provide a range of vitamins, minerals, and antioxidants that are important for menopausal women.

- The lemon juice and oregano in the marinade add flavor and may also have anti•inflammatory properties. Grilling the skewers is a healthy cooking method that preserves the nutrients in the ingredients.

60. Zucchini Noodles with Pesto and Cherry Tomatoes

Ingredient:

For the Zucchini Noodles:
• 3 medium zucchini, spiralized or julienned
• 1 tbsp olive oil

For the Toppings:
• 1 cup cherry tomatoes, halved
• 2 tbsp toasted pine nuts
• Grated Parmesan cheese (optional)

For the Pesto:
• 2 cups fresh basil leaves
• 1/4 cup pine nuts
• 2 cloves garlic
• 1/4 cup grated Parmesan cheese
• 2 tbsp olive oil
• 1 tbsp lemon juice
• Salt and pepper to taste

Instructions:

1. Make the zucchini noodles: Using a spiralizer, julienne slicer, or vegetable peeler, cut the zucchini into long, thin noodle•like strips. Set aside.

2. Make the pesto: In a food processor or blender, combine the basil, 1/4 cup pine nuts, garlic, Parmesan, olive oil, and lemon juice. Blend until a smooth pesto forms. Season with salt and pepper to taste.

3. In a large skillet, heat the 1 tbsp of olive oil over medium heat. Add the zucchini noodles and sauté for 2•3 minutes, just until they start to soften slightly. Be careful not to overcook them.

4. Remove the skillet from the heat and toss the zucchini noodles with the prepared pesto until evenly coated.

5. Transfer the pesto•coated zucchini noodles to a serving bowl or plate. Top with the halved cherry tomatoes, toasted pine nuts, and additional Parmesan cheese, if desired.

This zucchini noodle dish is an excellent choice for women during menopause for several reasons:

• Zucchini is a low•calorie, high•fiber vegetable that can help support digestive health. The pesto is made with nutrient•rich basil, which contains antioxidants that may help reduce inflammation.

• Pine nuts are a good source of healthy fats, protein, and minerals like magnesium and zinc, which are important during menopause.

• Cherry tomatoes provide a burst of flavor and are rich in vitamins, such as vitamin C, which can help support the immune system.

61. Almond Butter and Apple Slices

Ingredient:

• 2 tablespoons almond butter
• 1 medium apple, cored and sliced

Instructions:

1. Wash and slice the apple into thin, bite•sized pieces.

2. Spread the almond butter evenly onto the apple slices.

Why this is a good menopause snack:

• Almonds and almond butter are a good source of healthy fats, protein, fiber, and magnesium • all of which can help manage some menopausal symptoms. The healthy fats and protein provide sustained energy.

• Apples are a good source of fiber, which can help with digestive issues that are common during menopause. They also contain antioxidants that may help reduce inflammation.

• This snack is low in sugar and carbs, which can help stabilize blood sugar levels and energy during menopause.

The combination of the creamy almond butter and crisp apple slices makes for a satisfying, nutritious snack that may help ease certain menopausal symptoms. Feel free to adjust the portion sizes as needed.

62. Hummus with Carrot and Cucumber Sticks

Ingredient:

- 1/4 tsp ground cumin
- 1/4 tsp paprika
- Salt and pepper to taste
- 2 medium carrots, peeled and cut into sticks
- 1 English cucumber, cut into sticks
- 1 (15 oz) can chickpeas (garbanzo beans), rinsed and drained
- 2 tbsp tahini (sesame seed paste)
- 2 tbsp fresh lemon juice
- 2 cloves garlic, minced
- 2 tbsp olive oil

Instructions:

1. In a food processor or high•powered blender, combine the rinsed and drained chickpeas, tahini, lemon juice, minced garlic, olive oil, cumin, and paprika. Process until smooth and creamy, scraping down the sides as needed.

2. Season the hummus with salt and pepper to taste.

3. Transfer the hummus to a serving bowl or plate. Arrange the carrot and cucumber sticks around the hummus, making it easy for dipping.

This hummus and veggie stick snack is an excellent choice for women during menopause for several reasons:

1. Hummus:
   • Chickpeas, the main ingredient in hummus, are a great source of plant•based protein, fiber, and complex carbohydrates, which can help provide sustained energy.
   • Tahini, a key component of hummus, is rich in calcium, which is important for bone health during menopause.

2. Carrots and Cucumbers:
   • Carrots are a good source of beta•carotene, an antioxidant that may help reduce the risk of certain types of cancer and support eye health.
   • Cucumbers are high in water content and provide hydration, which can be beneficial during menopause when dehydration is more common.

3. Overall Nutrition: This snack is low in calories, high in fiber, and provides a balance of nutrients that can support overall health and well•being during menopause.

Enjoy this simple, nutritious, and satisfying snack as a healthy option during your menopausal journey.

63. Greek Yogurt with Honey and Walnuts

Ingredient:

• 1 cup plain Greek yogurt
• 1•2 tablespoons honey
• 2 tablespoons chopped walnuts

Instructions:

1. Spoon the Greek yogurt into a bowl.

2. Drizzle the honey over the yogurt.

3. Sprinkle the chopped walnuts on top.

Why this is a good option for menopause:

• Greek yogurt is an excellent source of protein, which can help maintain muscle mass and bone health during menopause.

• Honey contains natural antioxidants and may help alleviate some menopausal symptoms like hot flashes.

• Walnuts are rich in omega•3 fatty acids, which can help reduce inflammation and support brain health.

This simple, nutrient•dense snack or light meal provides a balance of protein, healthy fats, and natural sweetness to support women's health during the menopausal transition. The combination of Greek yogurt, honey, and walnuts makes for a delicious and satisfying treat.

64. Edamame with Sea Salt

Ingredient:

• 1 lb frozen edamame in the pod
• 1•2 tsp coarse sea salt

Instructions:

1. Bring a large pot of water to a boil over high heat.

2. Add the frozen edamame pods to the boiling water and cook for 5•7 minutes, or until the pods are bright green and tender.

3. Drain the cooked edamame in a colander and transfer them to a serving bowl.

4. Sprinkle the cooked edamame with the coarse sea salt, to taste. Start with 1 tsp of salt and add more if desired.

5. Serve the edamame warm or at room temperature.

This simple edamame snack is an excellent choice for women during menopause for several reasons:

1. Edamame:
   • Edamame is a type of immature soybean that is rich in plant•based protein, fiber, and a variety of vitamins and minerals.

   • Soy•based foods like edamame may help alleviate some menopausal symptoms, such as hot flashes and night sweats, due to their phytoestrogen content.

2. Sea Salt:
   • Sea salt is a minimally processed salt that contains trace minerals, which can help replenish electrolytes and support overall health.

   • The crunchy texture and savory flavor of the sea salt complement the edamame perfectly.

Edamame is a convenient, portable, and nutrient•dense snack that can be enjoyed on its own or as part of a larger meal. It's a great option for women during menopause who are looking for a healthy, satisfying, and easy•to•prepare snack.

65. Mixed Nuts and Dried Fruit

Ingredient:

- 1 cup mixed nuts (such as almonds, cashews, pecans, walnuts)
- 1/2 cup dried fruit (such as cranberries, apricots, figs, raisins)
- 1 tbsp honey (optional)
- 1 tsp ground cinnamon (optional)
- 1/4 tsp sea salt (optional)

Instructions:

1. In a medium bowl, combine the mixed nuts and dried fruit.

2. If desired, drizzle the honey over the nut and fruit mixture and toss to coat evenly.

3. Sprinkle the cinnamon and salt (if using) over the top and toss again to distribute.

4. Serve the mixed nuts and dried fruit as a snack or appetizer. You can also use it as a topping for yogurt, oatmeal, or salads.

5. Store any leftovers in an airtight container at room temperature for up to 1 week.

The combination of crunchy nuts and chewy dried fruit makes this a tasty and nutritious snack. The honey and spices are optional but add a nice touch of sweetness and warmth. Adjust the ingredients to your taste preferences.

66. Roasted Chickpeas

Ingredient:

• 1 (15 oz) can chickpeas (garbanzo beans), drained and rinsed
• 1 tbsp olive oil
• 1 tsp ground cumin
• 1 tsp paprika
• 1/2 tsp garlic powder
• 1/4 tsp cayenne pepper (optional, for a spicy kick)
• 1/4 tsp salt

Instructions:

1. Preheat your oven to 400°F (200°C).

2. Pat the drained and rinsed chickpeas dry with a paper towel or clean kitchen towel. This helps them get crispy when roasted.

3. In a medium bowl, toss the chickpeas with the olive oil, cumin, paprika, garlic powder, cayenne (if using), and salt until evenly coated.

4. Spread the seasoned chickpeas in a single layer on a baking sheet lined with parchment paper.

5. Roast for 20•25 minutes, shaking the pan halfway, until the chickpeas are crispy and lightly browned.

6. Allow the roasted chickpeas to cool slightly before serving. They can be enjoyed as a snack or added to salads, soups, or other dishes.

Why are roasted chickpeas beneficial for menopause?

• Chickpeas are a good source of plant•based protein, fiber, and complex carbohydrates, which can help manage blood sugar levels.

• They contain isoflavones, a type of phytoestrogen that can help alleviate menopausal symptoms like hot flashes and night sweats.

• The spices used, like cumin and paprika, have anti•inflammatory properties that may help reduce menopausal discomfort.

Enjoy these crispy, flavorful roasted chickpeas as a healthy snack during menopause!

67. Cottage Cheese with Cherry Tomatoes

Ingredient:

- 1 cup low•fat or non•fat cottage cheese
- 1 cup cherry tomatoes, halved
- 1 tbsp chopped fresh basil (or 1 tsp dried basil)
- 1 tsp extra•virgin olive oil
- Salt and pepper to taste

Instructions:

1. In a small bowl, combine the cottage cheese, halved cherry tomatoes, chopped fresh basil (or dried basil), and olive oil.

2. Gently stir the ingredients together until well combined.

3. Season with salt and pepper to taste. Serve immediately or refrigerate until ready to enjoy.

This simple dish is an excellent choice for women during menopause for several reasons:

1. Cottage Cheese:
   - Cottage cheese is a great source of protein, which can help maintain muscle mass and support overall health during menopause.
   - It's also a good source of calcium, which is important for bone health as estrogen levels decline during this transition.

2. Cherry Tomatoes:
   - Cherry tomatoes are rich in antioxidants, such as lycopene, which may help reduce the risk of certain health conditions associated with menopause.
   - They also provide vitamins C and K, which are important for immune function and bone health.

3. Basil and Olive Oil:
   - Basil contains anti•inflammatory properties that may help alleviate some of the symptoms associated with menopause, such as joint pain.
   - Olive oil is a healthy fat that can help support cardiovascular health and reduce the risk of chronic diseases.

This dish is easy to prepare, nutrient•dense, and can be enjoyed as a snack or a light meal. It's a great way to incorporate some of the key nutrients that are important for women during menopause.

68. Dark Chocolate and Almonds

Ingredient:

• 1 cup raw almonds
• 4 oz dark chocolate, chopped or broken into pieces

Instructions:

1. Preheat your oven to 350°F (175°C).

2. Spread the raw almonds in a single layer on a baking sheet. Toast the almonds in the preheated oven for 8•10 minutes, stirring halfway, until fragrant and lightly browned.

3. Remove the toasted almonds from the oven and let them cool completely.

4. In a small bowl, combine the toasted almonds and the chopped dark chocolate. Gently toss to mix.

5. Serve the dark chocolate and almonds as a snack. You can also store any leftovers in an airtight container at room temperature for up to 1 week.

Tips:
• Use high•quality dark chocolate with a cocoa content of 70% or higher for maximum health benefits.

• You can also add a pinch of sea salt to the mixture for a sweet and salty flavor.

• For a festive touch, you can drizzle a small amount of melted dark chocolate over the almonds.

This simple combination of dark chocolate and toasted almonds makes for a delicious and nutritious snack. The almonds provide healthy fats, protein, and fiber, while the dark chocolate is rich in antioxidants and can help satisfy sweet cravings.

69. Fresh Fruit Salad

Ingredient:

- 1 cup diced pineapple
- 1 cup diced mango
- 1 cup diced strawberries
- 1 cup diced kiwi
- 1 cup diced grapes
- 1 tbsp fresh lime juice
- 1 tbsp honey (optional)
- 1/4 tsp ground cinnamon (optional)

Instructions:

1. In a large bowl, combine the diced pineapple, mango, strawberries, kiwi, and grapes.

2. Drizzle the lime juice over the fruit and gently toss to coat.

3. If desired, drizzle the honey over the fruit salad and sprinkle the ground cinnamon on top. Gently toss to combine.

4. Cover the fruit salad and refrigerate for at least 30 minutes to allow the flavors to meld.

5. Serve the fresh fruit salad chilled, as a side dish or a refreshing snack.

Variations:

- You can use any combination of your favorite fresh fruits, such as berries, citrus, melon, etc.

- Add a splash of orange juice or a teaspoon of vanilla extract for extra flavor.

- For a creamy fruit salad, fold in a dollop of plain Greek yogurt or whipped cream.

- Sprinkle toasted nuts, shredded coconut, or a pinch of ground ginger on top.

This vibrant and colorful fruit salad is a great way to enjoy the natural sweetness and nutrition of fresh seasonal fruits. It's a refreshing and healthy option for a snack, dessert, or side dish.

70. Avocado and Tomato on Whole Grain Crackers

Ingredient:

• 1 ripe avocado, mashed
• 1 cup cherry or grape tomatoes, halved
• 1 tbsp fresh lemon juice
• 1 tbsp chopped fresh basil (or 1 tsp dried basil)
• Salt and pepper to taste
• 8•10 whole grain crackers

Instructions:

1. In a small bowl, mash the avocado with a fork until it's creamy and smooth.

2. Add the halved tomatoes, lemon juice, and chopped fresh basil (or dried basil). Gently stir to combine.

3. Season the avocado•tomato mixture with salt and pepper to taste. Spread the avocado•tomato mixture evenly onto the whole grain crackers. Serve the avocado and tomato crackers immediately.

This snack is an excellent choice for women during menopause for several reasons:

1. Avocado:
  • Avocados are a great source of healthy monounsaturated fats, which can help support heart health and reduce the risk of chronic diseases.
   • They also contain fiber, vitamins, and minerals that are important for overall well•being during menopause.

2. Tomatoes:
   • Tomatoes are rich in the antioxidant lycopene, which may help reduce the risk of certain types of cancer and cardiovascular disease.
   • They also provide vitamins C and K, which are important for immune function and bone health.

3. Whole Grain Crackers:
   • Whole grain crackers are a good source of complex carbohydrates, which can provide sustained energy and help maintain blood sugar levels.
   • They also contain fiber, which can support digestive health and help manage menopausal symptoms like constipation.

This simple and delicious snack is a great way to incorporate healthy fats, antioxidants, and fiber into your diet during menopause. The combination of creamy avocado, juicy tomatoes, and crunchy whole grain crackers makes for a satisfying and nutritious treat.

71. Rice Cakes with Peanut Butter and Banana

Ingredient:

- 2 whole grain rice cakes
- 2 tbsp natural peanut butter
- 1 small ripe banana, sliced
- 1 tsp honey (optional)
- Cinnamon (optional)

Instructions:

1. Spread the peanut butter evenly over the rice cakes.

2. Arrange the sliced banana on top of the peanut butter.

3. If desired, drizzle the honey over the banana slices. Sprinkle a light dusting of cinnamon over the top (optional).

Why is this snack beneficial for menopause?

- Whole grain rice cakes provide complex carbohydrates, which can help maintain stable blood sugar levels.

- Peanut butter is a good source of protein, healthy fats, and magnesium, all of which are important during menopause.

- Bananas are rich in potassium, which can help regulate blood pressure and reduce the risk of osteoporosis.

- Honey contains antioxidants and may help alleviate menopausal symptoms like hot flashes and night sweats.

- Cinnamon has anti•inflammatory properties and may help manage blood sugar levels.

This simple, nutrient•dense snack can provide a satisfying and energizing boost during the menopausal transition. The combination of complex carbs, protein, healthy fats, and beneficial plant compounds can help support overall health and well•being.

Feel free to adjust the ingredients to your taste preferences. You can also try using other nut or seed butters in place of peanut butter.

72. Baked Kale Chips

Ingredient:

• 1 bunch of kale, stems removed and leaves torn into bite•sized pieces
• 1 tbsp olive oil
• 1/4 tsp salt
• 1/8 tsp black pepper

Instructions:

1. Preheat your oven to 325°F (165°C).

2. Wash the kale leaves and pat them dry thoroughly with paper towels or a clean kitchen towel. This is important to ensure the kale chips get crispy.

3. In a large bowl, toss the kale leaves with the olive oil, salt, and black pepper until the leaves are evenly coated.

4. Spread the kale leaves in a single layer on a large baking sheet lined with parchment paper.

5. Bake for 12•15 minutes, flipping the kale leaves halfway through, until they are crispy and lightly browned.

6. Remove the baked kale chips from the oven and let them cool completely before serving.

Tips:
• For extra flavor, try sprinkling the kale with garlic powder, onion powder, or a pinch of cayenne pepper before baking.

• You can also experiment with different types of kale, such as curly kale, lacinato kale, or red kale.

• Store any leftover kale chips in an airtight container at room temperature for up to 5 days.

Kale is a nutrient•dense superfood that is packed with vitamins, minerals, and antioxidants. Baking it into crispy, flavorful chips is a delicious way to enjoy the health benefits of kale. These Baked Kale Chips make a great healthy snack or side dish.

73. Turkey and Cheese Roll•Ups

Ingredient:

• 8 slices of turkey breast, thinly sliced
• 4 slices of low•fat cheddar or Swiss cheese
• 1 tbsp Dijon mustard
• 1 tbsp chopped fresh parsley (optional)
• 1/4 tsp ground black pepper

Instructions:

1. Lay the turkey slices out flat on a clean work surface.

2. Place a slice of cheese on each turkey slice, leaving a small border around the edges.

3. Spread a thin layer of Dijon mustard over the cheese.

4. Sprinkle the chopped parsley (if using) and black pepper over the cheese.

5. Carefully roll up each turkey slice, starting from the short end and rolling tightly.

6. Secure the roll•ups with toothpicks or cut them in half diagonally to serve.

Why are these Turkey and Cheese Roll•Ups beneficial for menopause?

• Turkey is a lean protein source, which can help maintain muscle mass and bone health during menopause.

• Cheese provides calcium, which is important for maintaining strong bones as estrogen levels decline.

• Mustard contains compounds like glucosinolates that may help regulate hormone levels and alleviate menopausal symptoms.

• Parsley is a rich source of antioxidants and has anti•inflammatory properties that may help reduce menopausal discomfort.

These Turkey and Cheese Roll•Ups make for a quick, easy, and nutritious snack or light meal that can be beneficial for women during the menopausal transition. The combination of protein, calcium, and anti•inflammatory ingredients can help support overall health and well•being.

74. Smoothie Popsicles with Berries

Ingredient:

- 1 cup mixed berries (such as strawberries, blueberries, raspberries)
- 1 cup plain Greek yogurt
- 1/2 cup unsweetened almond milk
- 2 tbsp honey (or maple syrup)
- 1 tsp vanilla extract
- 1/4 tsp ground cinnamon

Instructions:

1. In a blender, combine the mixed berries, Greek yogurt, almond milk, honey, vanilla extract, and cinnamon. Blend until smooth.

2. Carefully pour the smoothie mixture into popsicle molds, leaving a small amount of space at the top for expansion.

3. Insert popsicle sticks and freeze the smoothie popsicles for at least 4 hours, or until completely frozen.

4. To remove the popsicles from the molds, run the molds under warm water for a few seconds, then gently pull the popsicles out.

Why are these Smoothie Popsicles beneficial for menopause?

- Berries are rich in antioxidants, which can help reduce inflammation and alleviate menopausal symptoms

- Greek yogurt provides protein, calcium, and probiotics, which are important for bone health and gut health during menopause.

- Almond milk is a good source of vitamin E, which can help manage hot flashes and night sweats.

- Honey and cinnamon have anti•inflammatory properties that may help reduce menopausal discomfort.

These refreshing Smoothie Popsicles are a delicious and healthy way to enjoy a nutrient•dense treat during the menopausal transition. The combination of fruits, dairy, and spices can provide a boost of essential nutrients and potentially help manage menopausal symptoms.

75. Trail Mix with Nuts and Seeds

Ingredient:

- 1 cup raw almonds
- 1 cup raw cashews
- 1/2 cup raw pumpkin seeds (pepitas)
- 1/2 cup raw sunflower seeds
- 1/2 cup unsweetened dried cranberries
- 1/4 cup unsweetened shredded coconut
- 1 tbsp chia seeds
- 1 tbsp ground flaxseeds
- 1/4 tsp ground cinnamon (optional)
- 1/8 tsp sea salt (optional)

Instructions:

1. In a large bowl, combine the almonds, cashews, pumpkin seeds, sunflower seeds, dried cranberries, shredded coconut, chia seeds, and ground flaxseeds.

2. If desired, sprinkle the ground cinnamon and sea salt over the mixture and stir to combine.

3. Transfer the trail mix to an airtight container or resealable bag. Store at room temperature for up to 2 weeks.

Variations:

- Swap in different nuts and seeds based on your preferences, such as pecans, walnuts, or hemp seeds.

- Add a small amount of dark chocolate chips or cacao nibs for a touch of sweetness.

- For a savory twist, toss in a teaspoon of smoked paprika or garlic powder.

- Use dried fruit like apricots, figs, or raisins instead of cranberries.

This homemade trail mix is a great source of healthy fats, protein, fiber, and essential vitamins and minerals. It's perfect for snacking, hiking, or adding to yogurt, oatmeal, or salads. The combination of nuts, seeds, and dried fruit provides a satisfying and nutrient•dense boost of energy.

76. Steamed Broccoli with Lemon

Ingredient:

• 1 lb fresh broccoli florets
• 2 tbsp water
• 1 tbsp fresh lemon juice
• 1 tsp olive oil
• 1/4 tsp salt
• 1/8 tsp black pepper

Instructions:

1. In a steamer basket set over a pot of simmering water, steam the broccoli florets for 5•7 minutes, until tender•crisp.

2. Carefully transfer the steamed broccoli to a serving bowl.

3. In a small bowl, whisk together the lemon juice, olive oil, salt, and black pepper.

4. Drizzle the lemon dressing over the hot broccoli and toss gently to coat.

5. Serve the Steamed Broccoli with Lemon warm, as a side dish.

Variations:

• For extra flavor, you can add a clove of minced garlic to the lemon dressing.

• Sprinkle the broccoli with a bit of grated lemon zest for a bright, citrusy note.

• Top the broccoli with toasted sliced almonds or grated Parmesan cheese.

• Use the lemon•dressed broccoli as a base for a salad or grain bowl.

This simple preparation allows the fresh, natural flavor of the broccoli to shine, while the lemon dressing adds a refreshing and tangy touch. Steaming the broccoli helps retain its nutrients and vibrant green color.

Broccoli is an excellent source of fiber, vitamins, and antioxidants, making it a great addition to a healthy diet. The lemon juice in this recipe also provides a boost of vitamin C.

77. Roasted Brussels Sprouts with Balsamic Glaze

Ingredient:

• 1 lb Brussels sprouts, trimmed and halved
• 2 tbsp olive oil
• 1/4 tsp salt
• 1/8 tsp black pepper
• 2 tbsp balsamic vinegar
• 1 tbsp honey

Instructions:

1. Preheat your oven to 400°F (200°C).

2. In a large bowl, toss the trimmed and halved Brussels sprouts with the olive oil, salt, and black pepper until the sprouts are evenly coated.

3. Spread the seasoned Brussels sprouts in a single layer on a baking sheet lined with parchment paper.

4. Roast the Brussels sprouts for 20•25 minutes, tossing halfway, until they are tender and lightly browned.

5. In a small saucepan, combine the balsamic vinegar and honey. Bring the mixture to a simmer over medium heat, stirring occasionally, until it thickens into a glaze, about 3•5 minutes.

6. Remove the roasted Brussels sprouts from the oven and drizzle the balsamic glaze over them, tossing to coat evenly. Serve the Roasted Brussels Sprouts with Balsamic Glaze warm, as a side dish.

Why are these Brussels sprouts beneficial for menopause?
• Brussels sprouts are a cruciferous vegetable that contains compounds like indole•3•carbinol, which can help regulate estrogen levels and alleviate menopausal symptoms.

• Balsamic vinegar is rich in antioxidants and may help reduce inflammation, which can be beneficial during menopause. Honey has anti•inflammatory properties and may help manage hot flashes and night sweats.

This flavorful and nutritious side dish of Roasted Brussels Sprouts with Balsamic Glaze can be a great addition to a menopausal woman's diet. The combination of cruciferous vegetables, vinegar, and honey provides a boost of beneficial nutrients and compounds that may help support overall health and well•being during the menopausal transition.

78. Quinoa Pilaf with Herbs

Ingredient:

- 1 cup uncooked quinoa, rinsed
- 2 cups low•sodium vegetable or chicken broth
- 1 tbsp olive oil
- 1 small onion, diced
- 2 cloves garlic, minced
- 1/2 cup diced bell pepper (any color)
- 1/4 cup chopped fresh parsley
- 2 tbsp chopped fresh basil
- 1 tbsp chopped fresh thyme
- 1/4 tsp salt
- 1/8 tsp black pepper

Instructions:

1. In a medium saucepan, combine the rinsed quinoa and broth. Bring the mixture to a boil over high heat.

2. Once boiling, reduce the heat to low, cover the saucepan, and simmer for 15•20 minutes, until the quinoa is tender and the liquid is absorbed.

3. In a large skillet, heat the olive oil over medium heat. Add the diced onion and sauté for 3•4 minutes, until translucent.

4. Add the minced garlic and diced bell pepper to the skillet. Cook for an additional 2•3 minutes, until fragrant.

5. Fluff the cooked quinoa with a fork and add it to the skillet with the sautéed vegetables. Stir to combine.

6. Remove the skillet from heat and stir in the chopped parsley, basil, and thyme. Season with salt and black pepper. Serve the Quinoa Pilaf with Herbs warm, as a side dish or a vegetarian main course.

Why is this recipe beneficial for menopause?

• Quinoa is a gluten•free, high•protein grain that can help maintain muscle mass and bone health during menopause.

• Herbs like parsley, basil, and thyme are rich in antioxidants and have anti•inflammatory properties that may help reduce menopausal discomfort.

• The bell peppers provide a boost of vitamin C, which can support immune function during the menopausal transition.

This flavorful and nutrient•dense Quinoa Pilaf with Herbs is a great option for women looking to incorporate more wholesome, menopause•friendly foods into their diet.

79. Cauliflower Rice with Cilantro

Ingredient:

• 1 medium head of cauliflower, cut into florets
• 2 tbsp olive oil
• 2 cloves garlic, minced
• 1/2 cup chopped fresh cilantro
• 1 tbsp fresh lime juice
• 1/4 tsp ground cumin
• 1/4 tsp salt
• 1/8 tsp black pepper

Instructions:

1. In a food processor, pulse the cauliflower florets in batches until they are broken down into small, rice•like pieces. Be careful not to over•process.

2. In a large skillet, heat the olive oil over medium heat. Add the minced garlic and sauté for 1 minute, until fragrant.

3. Add the riced cauliflower to the skillet and cook, stirring occasionally, for 5•7 minutes until the cauliflower is tender and lightly browned.

4. Remove the skillet from heat and stir in the chopped cilantro, lime juice, cumin, salt, and black pepper. Toss to combine.

5. Serve the Cauliflower Rice with Cilantro warm, as a side dish or a base for other dishes.

Why is this recipe beneficial for menopause?

• Cauliflower is a cruciferous vegetable that contains compounds like indole•3•carbinol, which can help regulate estrogen levels and alleviate menopausal symptoms.

• Cilantro is a herb rich in antioxidants and has anti•inflammatory properties that may help reduce menopausal discomfort.

• The lime juice provides a boost of vitamin C, which can support immune function during menopause.

• The cumin and black pepper in this dish have thermogenic properties that may help manage hot flashes.

This flavorful Cauliflower Rice with Cilantro is a nutritious and versatile side dish that can be a great addition to a menopausal woman's diet.

80. Sweet Potato Fries (baked)

Ingredient:

• 2 lbs sweet potatoes, peeled and cut into 1/2•inch thick fry shapes
• 2 tbsp olive oil
• 1 tsp ground cinnamon
• 1/2 tsp garlic powder
• 1/4 tsp salt
• 1/8 tsp black pepper

Instructions:

1. Preheat your oven to 400°F (200°C). Line a large baking sheet with parchment paper.

2. In a large bowl, toss the cut sweet potato fries with the olive oil, cinnamon, garlic powder, salt, and black pepper until the fries are evenly coated.

3. Spread the seasoned sweet potato fries in a single layer on the prepared baking sheet, making sure they are not touching each other.

4. Bake for 20•25 minutes, flipping the fries halfway through, until they are tender and lightly browned.

5. Remove the baked sweet potato fries from the oven and serve hot.

Why are these Sweet Potato Fries beneficial for menopause?

• Sweet potatoes are a rich source of beta•carotene, which can help regulate hormone levels and alleviate menopausal symptoms like hot flashes.

• The cinnamon in this recipe has anti•inflammatory properties that may help reduce menopausal discomfort.

• Garlic is a natural antioxidant that can support overall health and well•being during the menopausal transition.

These Baked Sweet Potato Fries are a healthier alternative to traditional french fries, providing a nutrient•dense and delicious side dish or snack. The combination of sweet potatoes, spices, and baking instead of frying makes this a great option for women looking to incorporate more menopause•friendly foods into their diet

81. Roasted Carrots with Thyme

Ingredient:

• 1 lb carrots, peeled and cut into 1•inch pieces
• 2 tbsp olive oil
• 1 tbsp fresh thyme leaves (or 1 tsp dried thyme)
• 1/2 tsp salt
• 1/4 tsp black pepper

Instructions:

1. Preheat your oven to 400°F (200°C). Line a baking sheet with parchment paper.

2. In a large bowl, toss the peeled and cut carrots with the olive oil, thyme, salt, and black pepper until the carrots are evenly coated.

3. Spread the seasoned carrots in a single layer on the prepared baking sheet.

4. Roast the carrots for 20•25 minutes, tossing halfway, until they are tender and lightly browned. Remove the roasted carrots from the oven and serve warm as a side dish.

Why are these Roasted Carrots with Thyme beneficial for menopause?

• Carrots are a rich source of beta•carotene, which can help regulate hormone levels and alleviate menopausal symptoms like hot flashes.

• Thyme is a herb with anti•inflammatory properties that may help reduce menopausal discomfort.

• The olive oil in this recipe provides healthy fats, which can help maintain skin and hair health during the menopausal transition.

This simple, flavorful side dish of Roasted Carrots with Thyme is a great way to incorporate more nutrient•dense, menopause•friendly foods into your diet. The combination of beta•carotene, anti•inflammatory herbs, and healthy fats can provide a range of benefits for women during the menopausal transition.

Feel free to adjust the amount of thyme or add other herbs like rosemary or oregano to suit your taste preferences.

82. Green Beans Almondine

Ingredient:

• 1 lb fresh green beans, trimmed
• 2 tbsp unsalted butter
• 1/3 cup sliced almonds
• 2 cloves garlic, minced
• 1 tbsp lemon juice
• 1/4 tsp salt
• 1/8 tsp black pepper

Instructions:

1. Bring a large pot of salted water to a boil. Add the trimmed green beans and cook for 4•6 minutes, until tender•crisp. Drain the beans and immediately transfer them to an ice bath to stop the cooking.

2. In a large skillet, melt the butter over medium heat. Add the sliced almonds and cook, stirring frequently, for 2•3 minutes until the almonds are lightly toasted.

3. Add the minced garlic to the skillet and cook for 1 minute, until fragrant.

4. Drain the chilled green beans and add them to the skillet with the toasted almonds and garlic. Toss to coat the beans evenly.

5. Drizzle the lemon juice over the green beans and season with salt and black pepper. Toss to combine. Serve the Green Beans Almondine warm, as a side dish.

Tips:

• For extra crunch, you can toast the almonds in a dry skillet before adding them to the recipe.

• Adjust the cooking time for the green beans based on your desired texture • less time for crisp•tender, more time for softer beans.

• You can also use slivered or sliced almonds instead of whole.

This simple yet elegant Green Beans Almondine dish features tender•crisp green beans tossed with toasted almonds, garlic, and a bright lemon flavor. It's a delicious and nutritious side that pairs well with a variety of main dishes.

83. Sautéed Spinach with Garlic

Ingredient:

• 1 lb fresh spinach, washed and stems removed
• 1 tbsp olive oil
• 3 cloves garlic, minced
• 1/4 tsp salt
• 1/8 tsp black pepper

Instructions:

1. In a large skillet or wok, heat the olive oil over medium heat.

2. Add the minced garlic to the hot oil and sauté for 1•2 minutes, until fragrant.

3. Gradually add the fresh spinach to the skillet, a few handfuls at a time, stirring constantly until the spinach is wilted down.

4. Once all the spinach has been added and wilted, season with salt and black pepper.

5. Continue to sauté the spinach for an additional 2•3 minutes, until it is tender. Serve the Sautéed Spinach with Garlic warm, as a side dish.

Why is this recipe beneficial for menopause?

• Spinach is a nutrient•dense leafy green that is rich in vitamins, minerals, and antioxidants, which can help support overall health during menopause.

• Garlic is a natural anti•inflammatory and can help regulate hormone levels, potentially reducing menopausal symptoms like hot flashes and night sweats.

• The olive oil in this dish provides healthy monounsaturated fats, which can help maintain skin and hair health as estrogen levels decline.

This simple, flavorful Sautéed Spinach with Garlic is a great way to incorporate more nutrient•dense, menopause•friendly greens into your diet. The combination of spinach, garlic, and olive oil can provide a range of potential benefits for women during the menopausal transition.

You can adjust the amount of garlic to your taste preferences, or try adding a squeeze of lemon juice or a sprinkle of red pepper flakes for extra flavor.

84. Grilled Asparagus with Olive Oil

Ingredient:

- 1 lb fresh asparagus, trimmed
- 2 tbsp olive oil
- 1 tbsp lemon juice
- 1 tsp garlic powder
- 1/4 tsp salt
- 1/8 tsp black pepper

Instructions:

1. Preheat your grill to medium•high heat.

2. In a large bowl, toss the trimmed asparagus spears with the olive oil, lemon juice, garlic powder, salt, and black pepper until the asparagus is evenly coated.

3. Arrange the seasoned asparagus in a single layer on the grill grates, perpendicular to the grates to prevent them from falling through.

4. Grill the asparagus for 5•7 minutes, turning occasionally, until they are tender and lightly charred. Remove the grilled asparagus from the grill and serve warm.

Why is this Grilled Asparagus with Olive Oil beneficial for menopause?

• Asparagus is a nutrient•dense vegetable that is rich in folate, which can help support overall health during the menopausal transition.

• Olive oil is a source of healthy monounsaturated fats, which can help maintain skin and hair health as estrogen levels decline.

• Garlic is a natural antioxidant that can support the immune system and reduce inflammation, which may help alleviate menopausal symptoms.

• Lemon juice provides a boost of vitamin C, which is important for maintaining bone health during menopause.

This simple, flavorful grilled asparagus dish is a great way to enjoy a seasonal vegetable that can also provide potential benefits for women going through menopause. The combination of asparagus, olive oil, and spices creates a delicious and nutritious side dish.

85. Wild Rice with Cranberries

Ingredient:

• 1 cup uncooked wild rice, rinsed
• 2 cups low•sodium vegetable or chicken broth
• 1/2 cup dried cranberries
• 2 tbsp chopped fresh parsley
• 1 tbsp olive oil
• 1 tsp lemon zest
• 1/4 tsp salt
• 1/8 tsp black pepper

Instructions:

1. In a medium saucepan, combine the rinsed wild rice and broth. Bring the mixture to a boil over high heat.

2. Once boiling, reduce the heat to low, cover the saucepan, and simmer for 45•50 minutes, until the rice is tender and the liquid is absorbed.

3. Remove the cooked wild rice from heat and fluff it with a fork.

4. Stir in the dried cranberries, chopped parsley, olive oil, lemon zest, salt, and black pepper until well combined. Serve the Wild Rice with Cranberries warm, as a side dish or a vegetarian main course.

Why is this recipe beneficial for menopause?
• Wild rice is a whole grain that is high in fiber, protein, and antioxidants, which can help support overall health during menopause.

• Cranberries are a rich source of polyphenols, which have anti•inflammatory properties that may help alleviate menopausal symptoms.

• Parsley is a herb that contains compounds like apigenin, which can help regulate hormone levels and reduce the risk of certain health issues associated with menopause.

• The lemon zest provides a boost of vitamin C, which can support immune function during the menopausal transition.

This flavorful and nutrient•dense Wild Rice with Cranberries dish is a great option for women looking to incorporate more wholesome, menopause•friendly foods into their diet. The combination of whole grains, antioxidants, and anti•inflammatory ingredients can provide a range of potential benefits.

86. Baked Zucchini Chips

Ingredient:

- 2 medium zucchinis, sliced into 1/4•inch thick rounds
- 1 tbsp olive oil
- 1 tsp garlic powder
- 1/2 tsp paprika
- 1/4 tsp salt
- 1/8 tsp black pepper

Instructions:

1. Preheat your oven to 400°F (200°C). Line two baking sheets with parchment paper.

2. In a large bowl, toss the sliced zucchini rounds with the olive oil, garlic powder, paprika, salt, and black pepper until the zucchini is evenly coated.

3. Arrange the seasoned zucchini slices in a single layer on the prepared baking sheets, making sure they are not overlapping.

4. Bake for 12•15 minutes, flipping the zucchini chips halfway, until they are crispy and lightly browned.

5. Remove the baked zucchini chips from the oven and let them cool slightly before serving.

Why are these Baked Zucchini Chips beneficial for menopause?

- Zucchini is a low•calorie, high•fiber vegetable that can help manage blood sugar levels and reduce the risk of heart disease during menopause.

- Garlic powder and paprika have anti•inflammatory properties that may help alleviate menopausal symptoms like hot flashes and joint pain.

- The olive oil in this recipe provides healthy monounsaturated fats, which can help maintain skin and hair health as estrogen levels decline.

These crispy, flavorful Baked Zucchini Chips make a great healthy snack or side dish. The combination of nutrient•dense zucchini, spices, and healthy fats can provide potential benefits for women going through the menopausal transition.

You can experiment with different seasoning blends, such as adding a pinch of cayenne pepper for a spicy kick or a sprinkle of grated Parmesan cheese for extra flavor.

87. Spicy Roasted Chickpeas

Ingredient:

- 1 (15 oz) can chickpeas, drained and rinsed
- 1 tbsp olive oil
- 1 tsp ground cumin
- 1 tsp paprika
- 1/2 tsp garlic powder
- 1/4 tsp cayenne pepper (or to taste)
- 1/4 tsp salt

Instructions:

1. Preheat your oven to 400°F (200°C). Line a baking sheet with parchment paper.

2. Pat the drained and rinsed chickpeas dry with a paper towel or clean kitchen towel.

3. In a medium bowl, toss the chickpeas with the olive oil, cumin, paprika, garlic powder, cayenne pepper, and salt until the chickpeas are evenly coated.

4. Spread the seasoned chickpeas in a single layer on the prepared baking sheet.

5. Roast the chickpeas for 20•25 minutes, shaking the pan halfway, until they are crispy and lightly browned. Remove the roasted chickpeas from the oven and let them cool slightly before serving.

Why are these Spicy Roasted Chickpeas beneficial for menopause?

• Chickpeas are a good source of plant•based protein, fiber, and complex carbohydrates, which can help manage blood sugar levels during menopause.

• The spices used, such as cumin and cayenne pepper, have anti•inflammatory properties that may help reduce menopausal discomfort. Garlic is a natural antioxidant that can support overall health and well•being during the menopausal transition.

These crispy, flavorful Spicy Roasted Chickpeas make a great snack or addition to salads and other dishes. The combination of protein, fiber, and spices can provide a nutritious boost for women going through menopause.

Feel free to adjust the amount of cayenne pepper to your desired level of spiciness. You can also experiment with other spice blends, such as adding a pinch of smoked paprika or chili powder.

88. Mashed Cauliflower

Ingredient:

• 1 large head of cauliflower, cut into florets
• 2 tbsp unsalted butter
• 2 tbsp plain Greek yogurt
• 1/4 cup unsweetened almond milk
• 1/2 tsp garlic powder
• 1/4 tsp salt
• 1/8 tsp black pepper

Instructions:

1. In a large pot, bring a few inches of water to a boil. Add the cauliflower florets, cover, and steam for 10•12 minutes, until very tender.

2. Drain the cooked cauliflower and transfer it to a food processor or high•powered blender.

3. Add the butter, Greek yogurt, almond milk, garlic powder, salt, and black pepper to the food processor.

4. Blend the ingredients together until the cauliflower is smooth and creamy, scraping down the sides as needed. Taste and adjust seasoning as desired. Serve the Mashed Cauliflower warm, as a side dish.

Why is this Mashed Cauliflower beneficial for menopause?
• Cauliflower is a cruciferous vegetable that contains compounds like indole•3•carbinol, which can help regulate estrogen levels and alleviate menopausal symptoms.

• Greek yogurt provides protein and probiotics, which can support gut health and overall well•being during the menopausal transition.

• Almond milk is a good source of vitamin E, which can help manage hot flashes and night sweats. Garlic is a natural antioxidant that can reduce inflammation and support the immune system.

This creamy, flavorful Mashed Cauliflower is a healthier alternative to traditional mashed potatoes. The combination of nutrient•dense cauliflower, protein•rich yogurt, and anti•inflammatory garlic can provide potential benefits for women going through menopause.

89. Couscous with Raisins and Almonds

Ingredient:

- 1 cup uncooked whole wheat couscous
- 1 cup boiling water
- 1/4 cup raisins
- 1/4 cup sliced almonds
- 2 tbsp olive oil
- 1 tbsp lemon juice
- 1 tsp ground cinnamon
- 1/4 tsp salt
- 1/8 tsp black pepper

Instructions:

1. In a medium bowl, combine the uncooked couscous and boiling water. Cover and let sit for 5•7 minutes, until the couscous has absorbed all the water.

2. Fluff the cooked couscous with a fork and stir in the raisins, sliced almonds, olive oil, lemon juice, cinnamon, salt, and black pepper.

3. Serve the Couscous with Raisins and Almonds warm or at room temperature, as a side dish or a light main course.

Why is this recipe beneficial for menopause?

• Whole wheat couscous is a complex carbohydrate that can help maintain stable blood sugar levels during menopause.

• Raisins are a good source of boron, a mineral that may help maintain bone health as estrogen levels decline.

• Almonds are rich in magnesium, which can help reduce the risk of osteoporosis and support overall health during the menopausal transition.

• Cinnamon has anti•inflammatory properties that may help alleviate menopausal symptoms like hot flashes and joint pain. Lemon juice provides a boost of vitamin C, which is important for immune function during menopause.

This flavorful and nutrient•dense Couscous with Raisins and Almonds dish is a great option for women looking to incorporate more wholesome, menopause•friendly foods into their diet. The combination of whole grains, dried fruit, nuts, and spices can provide a range of potential benefits.

90. Grilled Corn on the Cob

Ingredient:

• 4 ears of fresh corn, husks and silk removed
• 2 tbsp olive oil
• 1 tsp chili powder
• 1/2 tsp garlic powder
• 1/4 tsp salt
• 1/8 tsp black pepper

Instructions:

1. Preheat your grill to medium•high heat.

2. In a small bowl, mix together the olive oil, chili powder, garlic powder, salt, and black pepper.

3. Brush the seasoned oil mixture evenly over the corn cobs, making sure to coat all sides.

4. Place the prepared corn cobs directly on the grill grates. Grill for 12•15 minutes, turning occasionally, until the corn is tender and lightly charred.

5. Remove the grilled corn from the grill and serve hot, with any remaining seasoned oil drizzled over the top.

Why is this Grilled Corn on the Cob beneficial for menopause?

• Corn is a good source of fiber, which can help manage blood sugar levels and reduce the risk of heart disease during menopause.

• The chili powder contains capsaicin, which may help alleviate hot flashes and night sweats.

• Garlic is a natural antioxidant that can support overall health and well•being during the menopausal transition.

This simple, flavorful grilled corn dish is a great way to enjoy a seasonal summer vegetable that can also provide potential benefits for women going through menopause. The combination of spices and grilling adds a delicious depth of flavor to the corn.

91. Chia Seed Pudding with Coconut Milk

Ingredient:

- 1/4 cup chia seeds
- 1 cup unsweetened coconut milk
- 1 tbsp maple syrup (or honey)
- 1 tsp vanilla extract
- 1/4 tsp ground cinnamon
- 1/4 cup fresh berries (such as blueberries or raspberries)

Instructions:

1. In a medium bowl, whisk together the chia seeds, coconut milk, maple syrup (or honey), vanilla extract, and cinnamon until well combined.

2. Cover the bowl and refrigerate the chia seed pudding for at least 2 hours, or up to 4 days, stirring occasionally, until thickened.

3. When ready to serve, divide the chia seed pudding into individual serving bowls or glasses. Top each serving with a sprinkling of fresh berries.

Why is this Chia Seed Pudding with Coconut Milk beneficial for menopause?

- Chia seeds are a rich source of omega•3 fatty acids, which can help reduce inflammation and alleviate menopausal symptoms.

- Coconut milk is a good source of healthy fats, which can help maintain skin and hair health during the menopausal transition.

- Berries are high in antioxidants and may help regulate hormone levels, potentially reducing the risk of certain health issues associated with menopause.

- Cinnamon has anti•inflammatory properties that may help manage hot flashes and night sweats.

- Maple syrup or honey provide a natural sweetener, which can help satisfy cravings without spiking blood sugar levels.

This creamy, nutrient•dense Chia Seed Pudding with Coconut Milk is a delicious and satisfying breakfast or snack option for women during menopause. The combination of chia seeds, coconut milk, and berries can provide a range of potential benefits.

92. Dark Chocolate Avocado Mousse

Ingredient:

• 1 ripe avocado, pitted and flesh scooped out
• 1/4 cup unsweetened cocoa powder
• 1/4 cup maple syrup (or honey)
• 1/4 cup unsweetened almond milk
• 1 tsp vanilla extract
• 1/4 tsp ground cinnamon
• Pinch of sea salt

Instructions:

1. In a food processor or high•powered blender, combine the avocado flesh, cocoa powder, maple syrup, almond milk, vanilla extract, cinnamon, and sea salt.

2. Blend the ingredients together until the mixture is smooth and creamy, scraping down the sides as needed.

3. Divide the dark chocolate avocado mousse into individual serving bowls or ramekins.

4. Refrigerate the mousse for at least 30 minutes before serving to allow it to set. Serve chilled, garnished with a sprinkle of cinnamon or a few fresh berries, if desired.

Why is this Dark Chocolate Avocado Mousse beneficial for menopause?

• Avocados are a good source of healthy monounsaturated fats, which can help maintain skin and hair health during the menopausal transition.

• Dark chocolate is rich in antioxidants and may help regulate hormone levels, potentially reducing the risk of certain health issues associated with menopause.

• Cinnamon has anti•inflammatory properties that may help alleviate menopausal symptoms like hot flashes and joint pain.

• Maple syrup or honey provide a natural sweetener, which can help satisfy cravings without spiking blood sugar levels.

This creamy, indulgent Dark Chocolate Avocado Mousse is a delicious and nutritious dessert or snack option for women during menopause. The combination of healthy fats, antioxidants, and anti•inflammatory ingredients can provide potential benefits.

93. Baked Apples with Cinnamon and Nuts

Ingredient:

- 1 tsp ground cinnamon
- 1/4 tsp ground nutmeg
- 2 tbsp unsalted butter, softened
- 1/4 cup water or apple cider
- 4 medium•sized apples (such as Honeycrisp or Gala)
- 1/4 cup chopped walnuts or pecans
- 2 tbsp brown sugar (or maple syrup)

Instructions:

1. Preheat your oven to 375°F (190°C).

2. Core the apples, leaving the bottom intact, and place them in a baking dish.

3. In a small bowl, mix together the chopped nuts, brown sugar (or maple syrup), cinnamon, and nutmeg.

4. Stuff the nut mixture into the center of each apple, packing it in gently.

5. Dot the top of each apple with a small amount of the softened butter.

6. Pour the water or apple cider into the bottom of the baking dish. Bake the apples for 30•40 minutes, or until they are tender when pierced with a fork.

7. Serve the Baked Apples with Cinnamon and Nuts warm, with the cooking liquid spooned over the top.

Optional Toppings: Vanilla ice cream or whipped cream, Caramel sauce, Chopped toasted almonds or pecans

Why are these Baked Apples beneficial for menopause?

• Apples are a good source of fiber, which can help manage blood sugar levels during menopause. Nuts, such as walnuts and pecans, provide healthy fats and protein, which can help maintain muscle mass and bone health.

• Cinnamon and nutmeg have anti•inflammatory properties that may help alleviate menopausal symptoms like hot flashes and joint pain.

This comforting and nutrient•dense Baked Apples with Cinnamon and Nuts dish can be a delightful dessert or a satisfying snack for women during the menopausal transition. The combination of fruit, nuts, and spices provides a range of potential benefits.

94. Greek Yogurt with Honey and Berries

Ingredient:

• 1 cup plain Greek yogurt
• 1•2 tablespoons honey
• 1/2 cup mixed berries (such as blueberries, raspberries, blackberries)

Instructions:

1. Spoon the Greek yogurt into a bowl.

2. Drizzle the honey over the yogurt.

3. Top with the mixed berries.

4. Gently stir to combine.

Why this is a good option for menopause:

• Greek yogurt is an excellent source of protein, which can help maintain muscle mass and bone health during menopause.

• Honey provides natural sweetness and contains antioxidants that may help reduce inflammation.

• Berries are rich in vitamins, minerals, and antioxidants that can help support overall health during menopause.

The combination of protein, healthy carbs, and antioxidants in this simple dish makes it a nutritious and satisfying option for women going through menopause. The natural sweetness can also help curb sugar cravings that are common during this time.

95. Quinoa and Almond Flour Brownies

Ingredient:

• 1 cup cooked and cooled quinoa
• 1/2 cup almond flour
• 1/3 cup unsweetened cocoa powder
• 1/4 cup maple syrup
• 1/4 cup melted coconut oil
• 2 eggs
• 1 tsp vanilla extract
• 1/4 tsp salt
• 1/4 tsp baking soda

Instructions:

1. Preheat your oven to 350°F (175°C). Grease an 8x8 inch baking pan.

2. In a food processor, blend the cooked quinoa until it reaches a smooth, paste•like consistency.

3. In a medium bowl, whisk together the quinoa puree, almond flour, cocoa powder, maple syrup, melted coconut oil, eggs, vanilla extract, salt, and baking soda until well combined.

4. Pour the brownie batter into the prepared baking pan, smoothing the top with a spatula.

5. Bake for 20•25 minutes, or until a toothpick inserted in the center comes out clean. Allow the brownies to cool completely in the pan before cutting into squares.

Variations:
• For a richer flavor, add 1/4 cup of chopped dark chocolate or chocolate chips to the batter.

• Sprinkle the top of the brownies with a dusting of powdered sugar or a drizzle of melted dark chocolate. Use honey or agave syrup instead of maple syrup.

These Quinoa and Almond Flour Brownies are a healthier twist on a classic dessert. The quinoa and almond flour provide a boost of protein, fiber, and healthy fats, while the cocoa powder and maple syrup satisfy the chocolate craving. Enjoy these moist and fudgy brownies as a guilt•free treat.

96. Fresh Berry Salad with Mint

Ingredient:

- 2 cups mixed fresh berries (such as strawberries, blueberries, raspberries, blackberries)
- 1/4 cup fresh mint leaves, chopped
- 1 tbsp honey
- 1 tbsp fresh lemon juice
- 1/4 tsp lemon zest
- Pinch of salt

Instructions:

1. In a medium bowl, gently toss together the mixed berries and chopped mint leaves.

2. In a small bowl, whisk together the honey, lemon juice, lemon zest, and salt until well combined.

3. Drizzle the honey•lemon dressing over the berry•mint mixture and toss gently to coat.

4. Serve immediately or refrigerate until ready to serve. The salad is best enjoyed within a few hours of making it.

Enjoy this refreshing and flavorful berry salad! The mint adds a nice cooling element to balance the sweetness of the berries. It's a perfect light and healthy summer dessert or side dish.

97. Banana Ice Cream with Almond Butter

Ingredient:

• 4 ripe bananas, peeled and frozen
• 2 tbsp creamy almond butter
• 1 tsp vanilla extract
• 1/4 tsp cinnamon (optional)

Instructions:

1. In a food processor or high•powered blender, blend the frozen banana chunks until smooth and creamy, scraping down the sides as needed.

2. Add the almond butter, vanilla extract, and cinnamon (if using). Blend again until fully incorporated and the mixture is light and fluffy.

3. Serve immediately for a soft•serve consistency, or transfer to an airtight container and freeze for 2•3 hours for a firmer ice cream texture.

Why this is great for menopause:

• Bananas are a good source of potassium, which can help regulate blood pressure and reduce the risk of heart disease, a common concern during menopause.

• Almond butter provides healthy fats and protein, which can help stabilize blood sugar levels and keep you feeling full.

• Cinnamon is a natural anti•inflammatory that may help alleviate some menopausal symptoms like joint pain.

• This dessert is dairy•free, making it a great option for those who are lactose intolerant or prefer to avoid dairy during menopause.

Enjoy this creamy, nutrient•dense banana ice cream as a healthy and delicious treat to help support your body during the menopausal transition.

98. Dark Chocolate Covered Strawberries

Ingredient:

• 1 lb fresh strawberries, washed and patted dry
• 8 oz dark chocolate, chopped (at least 70% cacao)
• 1 tbsp coconut oil (optional)

Instructions:

1. Line a baking sheet with parchment paper or a silicone baking mat.

2. In a double boiler or a heatproof bowl set over a saucepan of simmering water, melt the dark chocolate, stirring occasionally, until smooth and fully melted. If using coconut oil, stir it in until well combined.

3. One at a time, hold the strawberries by the stem and dip them into the melted chocolate, coating them about 3/4 of the way up. Gently tap off any excess chocolate.

4. Place the chocolate•dipped strawberries on the prepared baking sheet, making sure they are not touching each other.. Refrigerate the strawberries for at least 30 minutes, or until the chocolate has fully set.

Why this is great for menopause:

• Dark chocolate is rich in antioxidants and may help reduce inflammation, which can alleviate some menopausal symptoms.

• Strawberries are a good source of vitamin C, which can help boost the immune system during menopause.

• The combination of dark chocolate and strawberries provides a delicious and satisfying treat that can help curb sweet cravings without the use of refined sugar.

• Coconut oil is a healthy fat that can help regulate hormone levels and support overall health during the menopausal transition.

Enjoy these decadent and nutritious dark chocolate covered strawberries as a guilt•free indulgence that can also provide some health benefits for women going through menopause.

99. Oatmeal Cookies with Raisins

Ingredient:

- 1 cup (2 sticks) unsalted butter, softened
- 1 cup brown sugar
- 1 egg
- 1 tsp vanilla extract

- 1 1/2 cups old•fashioned oats
- 1 1/4 cups all•purpose flour
- 1 tsp baking soda
- 1/2 tsp ground cinnamon
- 1/4 tsp salt
- 1 cup raisins

Instructions:

1. Preheat the oven to 350°F. Line two baking sheets with parchment paper.

2. In a large bowl, cream the softened butter and brown sugar together until light and fluffy, about 2•3 minutes. Beat in the egg and vanilla extract until well combined.

3. In a separate bowl, whisk together the oats, flour, baking soda, cinnamon, and salt.

4. Gradually add the dry ingredients to the wet ingredients, mixing just until combined. Fold in the raisins.

5. Scoop rounded tablespoons of dough onto the prepared baking sheets, spacing them about 2 inches apart.

6. Bake for 10•12 minutes, or until the edges are lightly golden brown. Allow the cookies to cool on the baking sheets for 5 minutes before transferring to a wire rack to cool completely.

Why this is great for menopause:

- Oats are a good source of fiber, which can help regulate digestion and reduce the risk of constipation, a common issue during menopause.

- Raisins are a natural source of phytoestrogens, which can help alleviate some menopausal symptoms like hot flashes and mood swings.

- Cinnamon is a natural anti•inflammatory that may help reduce joint pain and other menopausal discomforts.

- The combination of oats, raisins, and cinnamon provides a nutrient•dense and satisfying cookie that can help support overall health during the menopausal transition.

Enjoy these delicious and wholesome oatmeal cookies as a comforting treat that can also provide some health benefits for women going through menopause.

100. Coconut Macaroons

Ingredient:

• 3 large egg whites
• 1/2 cup granulated sugar
• 1/4 tsp salt
• 2 1/2 cups unsweetened shredded coconut
• 1 tsp vanilla extract

Instructions:

1. Preheat the oven to 325°F. Line a baking sheet with parchment paper.

2. In a medium bowl, beat the egg whites with an electric mixer until they are foamy and start to hold soft peaks.

3. Gradually add the sugar, 1 tablespoon at a time, while continuing to beat the egg whites until they form stiff, glossy peaks.

4. Gently fold in the salt, shredded coconut, and vanilla extract until well combined.

5. Scoop rounded tablespoons of the coconut mixture onto the prepared baking sheet, spacing them about 1 inch apart.

6. Bake for 18•20 minutes, or until the macaroons are lightly golden brown on the edges.

7. Remove the macaroons from the oven and let them cool on the baking sheet for 5 minutes before transferring to a wire rack to cool completely.

Why this is great for menopause:

• Coconut is a good source of healthy fats, which can help regulate hormone levels and reduce the risk of heart disease during menopause.

• Egg whites are a lean protein that can help maintain muscle mass and support overall health.

• Vanilla extract has a calming effect that may help alleviate some menopausal symptoms like mood swings and anxiety.

• These macaroons are naturally sweetened with sugar, providing a healthier alternative to processed sweets.

101. Mango Sorbet

Ingredient:

- 3 cups chopped ripe mango (about 3•4 mangoes)
- 1/2 cup water
- 1/4 cup honey or maple syrup
- 1 tbsp fresh lime juice
- 1/4 tsp ground ginger (optional)

Instructions:

1. In a blender or food processor, puree the chopped mango until smooth.

2. In a small saucepan, combine the water and honey/maple syrup. Heat over medium, stirring occasionally, until the sweetener has dissolved. Remove from heat and let cool completely.

3. Once the sweetener mixture is cooled, add it to the mango puree along with the lime juice and ground ginger (if using). Blend until well combined.

4. Pour the mango mixture into a shallow baking dish or metal pan and place in the freezer. Stir the mixture every 30 minutes for the first 2 hours, then every hour thereafter, until it reaches your desired sorbet consistency, about 3•4 hours total.

5. Scoop into bowls or cups and serve immediately. You can also transfer the sorbet to an airtight container and freeze for up to 2 months.

Why this is great for menopause:

- Mangoes are a good source of vitamin C, which can help boost the immune system during menopause.

- The natural sweetness from the honey or maple syrup provides a healthier alternative to refined sugar.

- Lime juice and ginger can help reduce inflammation, which may alleviate some menopausal symptoms.

- This sorbet is dairy•free, making it a great option for those who are lactose intolerant or prefer to avoid dairy during menopause.

Enjoy this refreshing and nutritious mango sorbet as a cool and satisfying treat to help support your body during the menopausal transition.

102. Almond Flour Chocolate Chip Cookies

Ingredient:

• 2 cups almond flour
• 1/2 tsp baking soda
• 1/4 tsp salt
• 1/2 cup unsalted butter, softened

• 1/2 cup granulated sweetener (such as erythritol or monk fruit sweetener)
• 1 egg
• 1 tsp vanilla extract
• 1/2 cup dark chocolate chips or chopped dark chocolate

Instructions:

1. Preheat the oven to 350°F. Line a baking sheet with parchment paper.

2. In a medium bowl, whisk together the almond flour, baking soda, and salt.

3. In a separate large bowl, beat the softened butter and granulated sweetener together until light and fluffy, about 2•3 minutes. Beat in the egg and vanilla extract until well combined.

4. Gradually add the dry ingredients to the wet ingredients, mixing just until combined. Fold in the dark chocolate chips.

5. Scoop rounded tablespoons of dough onto the prepared baking sheet, spacing them about 2 inches apart.

6. Bake for 12•15 minutes, or until the edges are lightly golden brown. Allow the cookies to cool on the baking sheet for 5 minutes before transferring to a wire rack to cool completely.

Why this is great for menopause:

• Almond flour is a low•carb, gluten•free flour that is high in healthy fats and protein, which can help regulate blood sugar levels and support overall health during menopause.

• Dark chocolate is rich in antioxidants and may help reduce inflammation, which can alleviate some menopausal symptoms.

• The use of a granulated sweetener like erythritol or monk fruit provides a healthier alternative to refined sugar, which can cause blood sugar spikes.

• These cookies are a satisfying and nutrient•dense treat that can help curb sweet cravings without the use of excessive sugar.

103. Baked Pears with Walnuts and Honey

Ingredient:

• 4 ripe but firm pears, halved and cored
• 1/4 cup chopped walnuts
• 2 tbsp honey
• 1 tsp ground cinnamon
• 1/4 tsp ground nutmeg
• Pinch of salt

Instructions:

1. Preheat the oven to 375°F. Line a baking sheet with parchment paper.

2. Arrange the pear halves, cut-side up, on the prepared baking sheet.

3. In a small bowl, mix together the chopped walnuts, honey, cinnamon, nutmeg, and a pinch of salt.

4. Spoon the walnut-honey mixture evenly into the center of each pear half.

5. Bake for 20-25 minutes, or until the pears are tender and the walnuts are lightly toasted. Remove the baked pears from the oven and let them cool for 5 minutes before serving.

Why this is great for menopause:

• Pears are a good source of fiber, which can help regulate digestion and reduce the risk of constipation, a common issue during menopause.

• Walnuts are rich in omega-3 fatty acids, which can help reduce inflammation and alleviate joint pain associated with menopause.

• Honey is a natural sweetener that can help satisfy cravings without the use of refined sugar, which can cause blood sugar spikes.

• Cinnamon and nutmeg are natural anti-inflammatory spices that may help alleviate some menopausal symptoms like hot flashes and mood swings.

Enjoy this warm, comforting, and nutrient-dense dessert as a healthy treat that can also provide some benefits for women going through menopause.

104. Protein Balls with Dates and Nuts

Ingredient:

• 1 cup raw almonds
• 1 cup raw walnuts
• 1 cup pitted Medjool dates
• 2 scoops (about 1/2 cup) vanilla protein powder
• 2 tbsp ground flaxseed
• 1 tsp ground cinnamon
• 1/4 tsp sea salt

Instructions:

1. In a food processor, pulse the almonds and walnuts until they are finely chopped, but not a powder.

2. Add the pitted dates, protein powder, ground flaxseed, cinnamon, and salt to the food processor. Pulse until the mixture is well combined and starts to stick together.

3. Scoop the mixture by the tablespoonful and roll into bite•sized balls with your hands.

4. Place the protein balls on a parchment•lined baking sheet and refrigerate for at least 30 minutes to allow them to firm up. Store the protein balls in an airtight container in the refrigerator for up to 1 week.

Why this is great for menopause:

• Nuts like almonds and walnuts are a good source of healthy fats, which can help regulate hormone levels and reduce the risk of heart disease during menopause.

• Dates are a natural sweetener that can help satisfy cravings without the use of refined sugar, which can cause blood sugar spikes.

• Protein powder helps maintain muscle mass and supports overall health during the menopausal transition.

• Flaxseed is rich in phytoestrogens, which may help alleviate some menopausal symptoms like hot flashes and mood swings.

• Cinnamon is a natural anti•inflammatory that may help reduce joint pain and other menopausal discomforts.

105. Lemon Blueberry Muffins

Ingredient:

- 2 cups all•purpose flour
- 1 tsp baking powder
- 1/2 tsp baking soda
- 1/4 tsp salt
- 1 cup fresh or frozen blueberries
- 1/2 cup unsalted butter, melted and slightly cooled
- 3/4 cup granulated sugar
- 2 large eggs
- 1 tsp vanilla extract
- 1 tbsp lemon zest
- 2 tbsp fresh lemon juice

Instructions:

1. Preheat the oven to 400°F. Grease a 12•cup muffin tin or line with paper liners.

2. In a medium bowl, whisk together the flour, baking powder, baking soda, and salt.

3. In a separate large bowl, whisk together the melted butter and sugar until combined. Beat in the eggs one at a time, then stir in the vanilla, lemon zest, and lemon juice.

4. Fold the dry ingredients into the wet ingredients just until combined, being careful not to overmix. Gently fold in the blueberries.

5. Divide the batter evenly among the prepared muffin cups, filling them about 3/4 full.

6. Bake for 18•20 minutes, or until a toothpick inserted in the center comes out clean.

7. Allow the muffins to cool in the tin for 5 minutes before transferring to a wire rack to cool completely.

Why this is great for menopause:

• Blueberries are rich in antioxidants and may help reduce inflammation, which can alleviate some menopausal symptoms.

• Lemon is a good source of vitamin C, which can help boost the immune system during menopause.

• The combination of lemon and blueberry provides a refreshing and flavorful muffin that can help satisfy sweet cravings without the use of excessive sugar.

• The healthy fats from the butter can help regulate hormone levels and support overall health during the menopausal transition.

Enjoy these delicious and nutritious lemon blueberry muffins as a tasty and comforting treat that can also provide some health benefits for women going through menopause.

106. Green Smoothie with Spinach and Pineapple

Ingredient:

• 1 cup unsweetened almond milk
• 1 cup fresh spinach leaves
• 1 cup frozen pineapple chunks
• 1 ripe banana, frozen
• 1 tbsp ground flaxseed
• 1 tsp honey (optional)

Instructions:

1. In a high•speed blender, combine the almond milk, spinach, pineapple, frozen banana, and ground flaxseed.

2. Blend on high speed until the mixture is smooth and creamy, about 1•2 minutes.

3. Taste the smoothie and add the honey if you'd like it to be a bit sweeter. Pour the green smoothie into a glass and enjoy immediately.

Why this is great for menopause:

• Spinach is a nutrient•dense green that is rich in vitamins, minerals, and antioxidants, which can help support overall health during menopause.

• Pineapple contains bromelain, an enzyme that may help reduce inflammation and alleviate joint pain associated with menopause.

• Bananas are a good source of potassium, which can help regulate blood pressure and reduce the risk of heart disease.

• Flaxseed is high in phytoestrogens, which may help alleviate some menopausal symptoms like hot flashes and mood swings.

• Almond milk is a dairy•free, low•calorie alternative that provides healthy fats to help regulate hormone levels.

• The natural sweetness from the pineapple and banana can help satisfy cravings without the use of refined sugar.

Enjoy this refreshing and nutrient•packed green smoothie as a healthy start to your day or a nourishing snack that can also provide some benefits for women going through menopause.

107. Turmeric Latte with Almond Milk

Ingredient:

• 2 cups unsweetened almond milk
• 1 tsp ground turmeric
• 1/2 tsp ground ginger
• 1/4 tsp ground cinnamon
• 1 tbsp honey (or maple syrup)
• Pinch of black pepper

Instructions:
1. In a small saucepan, whisk together the almond milk, turmeric, ginger, cinnamon, and black pepper.

2. Heat the mixture over medium heat, whisking frequently, until it starts to steam and bubble slightly, about 5 minutes. Do not let it boil.

3. Remove the saucepan from the heat and stir in the honey (or maple syrup) until well combined. Pour the turmeric latte into mugs and enjoy immediately.

Why this is great for menopause:
• Turmeric is a powerful anti•inflammatory spice that may help alleviate joint pain and other menopausal symptoms.

• Ginger also has anti•inflammatory properties and may help reduce nausea and digestive issues common during menopause.

• Cinnamon can help regulate blood sugar levels and may have a calming effect on the body.

• Almond milk is a dairy•free, low•calorie alternative that is rich in healthy fats, which can help support hormone balance.

• Honey or maple syrup provide a natural sweetener to balance the earthy flavors of the spices.

• The combination of these ingredients creates a comforting and nourishing beverage that can help support overall health during the menopausal transition.

Enjoy this soothing and flavorful turmeric latte as a warm and cozy drink that can also provide some health benefits for women going through menopause.

108. Herbal Tea with Lemon and Ginger

Ingredient:

• 4 cups water
• 2 tbsp dried herbal tea (such as chamomile, peppermint, or hibiscus)
• 1•inch piece of fresh ginger, peeled and sliced
• 1 lemon, sliced
• 1 tbsp honey (optional)

Instructions:
1. In a medium saucepan, bring the water to a boil.

2. Add the dried herbal tea and the sliced ginger to the boiling water. Reduce the heat and let the tea steep for 5•7 minutes.

3. Remove the saucepan from the heat and stir in the lemon slices.

4. Pour the tea into mugs, making sure to include some of the lemon and ginger slices.

5. If desired, stir in 1 tbsp of honey per mug to add a touch of sweetness. Serve the herbal tea hot and enjoy.

Why this is great for menopause:
• Chamomile, peppermint, and hibiscus teas have been shown to have anti•inflammatory properties, which can help alleviate some menopausal symptoms like joint pain and headaches.

• Ginger is a natural anti•inflammatory and may help reduce nausea and digestive issues common during menopause.

• Lemon is a good source of vitamin C, which can help boost the immune system and reduce inflammation.

• Honey is a natural sweetener that can help satisfy cravings without the use of refined sugar, which can cause blood sugar spikes.

• The combination of these ingredients creates a soothing and nourishing herbal tea that can help support overall health during the menopausal transition.

Enjoy this comforting and flavorful herbal tea as a warm and calming beverage that can provide some benefits for women going through menopause.

109. Berry Protein Shake

Ingredient:

- 1 cup unsweetened almond milk
- 1/2 cup frozen mixed berries (such as blueberries, raspberries, and blackberries)
- 1 scoop vanilla or berry•flavored protein powder
- 1 tbsp ground flaxseed
- 1 tsp honey (optional)

Instructions:

1. In a high•speed blender, combine the almond milk, frozen berries, protein powder, and ground flaxseed.

2. Blend on high speed until the mixture is smooth and creamy, about 1•2 minutes.

3. Taste the shake and add the honey if you'd like it to be a bit sweeter.

4. Pour the berry protein shake into a glass and enjoy immediately.

Why this is great for menopause:

- Berries are rich in antioxidants and may help reduce inflammation, which can alleviate some menopausal symptoms like joint pain and hot flashes.

- Protein powder helps maintain muscle mass and supports overall health during the menopausal transition.

- Almond milk is a dairy•free, low•calorie alternative that provides healthy fats to help regulate hormone levels.

- Flaxseed is a good source of fiber and phytoestrogens, which may help alleviate some menopausal symptoms like hot flashes and mood swings.

- The natural sweetness from the berries and optional honey can help satisfy cravings without the use of refined sugar.

Enjoy this nutrient•dense and satisfying berry protein shake as a healthy breakfast or snack that can also provide some benefits for women going through menopause.

110. Coconut Water with Fresh Mint

Ingredient:

• 4 cups unsweetened coconut water
• 10•12 fresh mint leaves
• 1 lime, sliced (optional)
• Ice cubes (optional)

Instructions:

1. In a pitcher or large glass, combine the coconut water and fresh mint leaves.

2. Stir the mixture well and let it sit for 5•10 minutes to allow the mint to infuse the coconut water.

3. Add the lime slices, if using, and stir again.

4. Pour the coconut water over ice cubes, if desired, and serve immediately.

Why this is great for menopause:

• Coconut water is a natural source of electrolytes, such as potassium, which can help regulate blood pressure and reduce the risk of heart disease during menopause.

• Mint has a cooling effect and may help alleviate some menopausal symptoms like hot flashes and digestive issues.

• Lime is a good source of vitamin C, which can help boost the immune system and reduce inflammation.

• This refreshing and hydrating beverage is a great alternative to sugary drinks, which can cause blood sugar spikes.

• The combination of coconut water, mint, and lime creates a flavorful and soothing drink that can help support overall health during the menopausal transition.

Enjoy this simple yet nourishing coconut water with fresh mint as a hydrating and rejuvenating drink throughout the day. It's a great way to stay hydrated and support your body during menopause.

111. Lemon and Cucumber Infused Water

Ingredient:

• 8 cups filtered water
• 1 lemon, sliced
• 1 cucumber, sliced
• 10•12 fresh mint leaves (optional)

Instructions:

1. In a large pitcher or water dispenser, combine the filtered water, lemon slices, and cucumber slices.

2. If using, add the fresh mint leaves to the pitcher as well.

3. Stir the mixture well and refrigerate for at least 2 hours, or up to 24 hours, to allow the flavors to infuse the water.

4. Serve the infused water chilled, making sure to include some of the fruit, vegetable, and mint (if using) in each glass. Refill the pitcher with more water as needed, and enjoy the infused water throughout the day.

Why this is a great option:

• Lemon is a good source of vitamin C, which can help boost the immune system and reduce inflammation.

• Cucumbers are hydrating and contain silica, which may help improve skin elasticity and reduce the appearance of wrinkles.

• Mint has a cooling effect and may help alleviate some menopausal symptoms like hot flashes and digestive issues.

• Infusing the water with these natural ingredients creates a refreshing and flavorful beverage that can encourage increased water intake.

• This infused water is a healthy and low•calorie alternative to sugary drinks, which can cause blood sugar spikes.

Enjoy this lemon and cucumber infused water as a hydrating and nourishing drink throughout the day. It's a great way to stay hydrated and support your overall health.

112. Almond Milk Smoothie with Chia Seeds

Ingredient:

• 1 cup unsweetened almond milk
• 1 frozen banana
• 1/2 cup frozen berries (such as blueberries, raspberries, or strawberries)
• 2 tbsp chia seeds
• 1 tbsp almond butter
• 1 tsp honey (optional)

Instructions:

1. In a high•speed blender, combine the almond milk, frozen banana, frozen berries, chia seeds, and almond butter.

2. Blend on high speed until the mixture is smooth and creamy, about 1•2 minutes.

3. Taste the smoothie and add the honey if you'd like it to be a bit sweeter. Pour the smoothie into a glass and enjoy immediately.

Why this is great for menopause:

• Almond milk is a dairy•free, low•calorie alternative that is rich in healthy fats, which can help regulate hormone levels during menopause.

• Bananas are a good source of potassium, which can help regulate blood pressure and reduce the risk of heart disease.

• Berries are high in antioxidants and may help reduce inflammation, which can alleviate some menopausal symptoms.

• Chia seeds are a great source of fiber, protein, and omega•3 fatty acids, all of which can support overall health during the menopausal transition.

• Almond butter provides additional healthy fats and protein to help keep you feeling full and satisfied.

• The natural sweetness from the banana and optional honey can help satisfy cravings without the use of refined sugar.

Enjoy this nutrient•dense and creamy smoothie as a healthy breakfast or snack that can also provide some benefits for women going through menopause.

113. Freshly Squeezed Orange Juice

Ingredient:

• 6•8 medium•sized oranges, washed

Instructions:

1. Cut the oranges in half crosswise.

2. Using a citrus juicer or a handheld juicer, squeeze the juice from the orange halves, collecting the juice in a pitcher or container.

3. Stir the juice to ensure it is well•mixed.

4. Pour the freshly squeezed orange juice into glasses and serve immediately.

Why this is great for menopause:

• Oranges are an excellent source of vitamin C, which can help boost the immune system and reduce inflammation during menopause.

• Vitamin C is also important for the production of collagen, which can help maintain skin elasticity and reduce the appearance of wrinkles.

• The natural sweetness of the orange juice can help satisfy cravings without the use of refined sugar, which can cause blood sugar spikes.

• Freshly squeezed orange juice is a hydrating and refreshing beverage that can help support overall health during the menopausal transition.

• Drinking orange juice can also help increase your intake of potassium, which is important for regulating blood pressure and reducing the risk of heart disease.

Enjoy this freshly squeezed orange juice as a healthy and delicious way to start your day or as a refreshing pick•me•up throughout the day. The natural nutrients and vitamins in the juice can provide valuable support for women going through menopause.

114. Matcha Green Tea Latte

Ingredient:

- 1 tsp matcha green tea powder
- 1 cup unsweetened almond milk
- 1 tbsp honey (or maple syrup)
- 1/2 tsp vanilla extract
- Pinch of ground cinnamon (optional)

Instructions:

1. In a small saucepan, whisk together the matcha powder and a small amount of the almond milk until the matcha is fully dissolved and there are no lumps.

2. Add the remaining almond milk to the saucepan and heat over medium, whisking frequently, until the mixture is steaming and hot but not boiling.

3. Remove the saucepan from the heat and stir in the honey (or maple syrup) and vanilla extract until well combined.

4. Pour the matcha latte into a mug and top with a sprinkle of ground cinnamon, if desired.

Why this is great for menopause:

- Matcha green tea is rich in antioxidants and may help reduce inflammation, which can alleviate some menopausal symptoms like joint pain and hot flashes.

- The caffeine in matcha can provide a gentle energy boost without the crash associated with coffee, which can be helpful during the menopausal transition.

- Almond milk is a dairy·free, low·calorie alternative that provides healthy fats to help regulate hormone levels.

- Honey or maple syrup offer a natural sweetener to balance the slightly bitter taste of the matcha, without the use of refined sugar.

- Cinnamon is a natural anti·inflammatory spice that may also have a calming effect on the body.

Enjoy this soothing and nourishing matcha green tea latte as a comforting and healthy beverage that can provide some benefits for women going through menopause.

115. Detox Water with Apple Cider Vinegar

Ingredient:

- 8 cups filtered water
- 2 tbsp raw, unfiltered apple cider vinegar
- 1 lemon, sliced
- 1 cucumber, sliced
- 10·12 fresh mint leaves

Instructions:

1. In a large pitcher, combine the filtered water, apple cider vinegar, lemon slices, cucumber slices, and mint leaves.

2. Stir the mixture well and refrigerate for at least 2 hours, or up to 24 hours, to allow the flavors to infuse the water.

3. Serve the detox water chilled, making sure to include some of the fruit, vegetable, and mint in each glass.

4. Refill the pitcher with more water as needed, and enjoy the detox water throughout the day.

Why this is great for menopause:

- Apple cider vinegar is believed to have detoxifying properties and may help regulate blood sugar levels, which can be beneficial during menopause.

- Lemons are a good source of vitamin C, which can help boost the immune system and reduce inflammation.

- Cucumbers are hydrating and contain silica, which may help improve skin elasticity and reduce the appearance of wrinkles.

- Mint has a cooling effect and may help alleviate some menopausal symptoms like hot flashes and digestive issues.

- The combination of these ingredients creates a refreshing and nourishing drink that can help support overall health during the menopausal transition.

Enjoy this detox water as a hydrating and flavorful alternative to plain water, and reap the potential benefits it can provide for women going through menopause.

Congratulations on exploring ***"The New Menopause Cookbook: Soothing Foods to Ease Menopause Symptoms With 115+ Recipes."*** We hope this journey through flavorful and nutritious recipes has brought you comfort, inspiration, and practical support during this transformative time in your life.

As you've discovered, food is not just sustenance but a powerful tool for managing menopausal symptoms and promoting overall well-being. By incorporating nutrient-rich ingredients and balanced meals into your diet, you've taken proactive steps to nourish your body and support hormonal balance. Whether it was finding relief from hot flashes with cooling salads, boosting energy levels with protein-packed dishes, or calming mood swings with soothing soups, each recipe was crafted with your health and happiness in mind.

Beyond the recipes, we hope this cookbook has empowered you with knowledge about how food can impact your menopause journey. From understanding the role of phytoestrogens to learning about the benefits of omega-3 fatty acids and antioxidants, you now have a toolbox of nutritional strategies to support your health for years to come.

Remember, your journey through menopause is unique, and so is your relationship with food. Continue to explore new flavors, adapt recipes to suit your preferences, and listen to your body's needs. Whether you're cooking for yourself, sharing meals with loved ones, or simply enjoying a quiet moment with a comforting dish, let food be a source of joy and healing.

Thank you for allowing us to be a part of your kitchen and health journey. May these recipes continue to nourish and empower you as you embrace this new chapter of life with strength, resilience, and delicious meals.

Wishing you good health and happiness always.

Bon appétit!